ScrubTales™ Registered Nurse

A Real World Career Guide That Tells the Truth About the Demands and Tradeoffs of Nursing

ScrubTales™ Series 1 — Core Clinical Careers

Mason Preddy

MASON MAISON
PUBLISHING™
REWRITING THE NARRATIVE
MASONMAISON.PUB

ScrubTales™: Registered Nurse

Published by

Mason Maison™ Publishing

masonmaison.pub

Printed in the United States of America.

Chapter 1

A Note to the Reader

Healthcare speaks its own language. As you move through this book, you may encounter clinical terms, acronyms, or professional vocabulary that may be unfamiliar, especially if you are early in your career exploration journey. To support clarity and learning, selected words throughout the text are marked with **(gl)**, indicating that the term appears in the glossary at the back of the book. These glossary references are designed to help you build professional vocabulary gradually while staying engaged with the larger career decision process.

Chapter 2

Welcome

Choosing to become a Registered Nurse is rarely a casual decision. It is a commitment to responsibility, to presence during moments that are often intense, uncertain, and deeply human. Yet many people enter nursing with only a partial understanding of what the work actually feels like day to day. Job descriptions explain duties. School programs teach skills. But very few resources help you understand how different nursing environments shape your identity, energy, and long-term sustainability in the profession. *ScrubTales™: Registered Nurse* exists to close that gap. This book is designed to help you see the real rhythms of nursing across specialties, understand how hiring systems actually work, and begin identifying where you are most likely to thrive—not just where you are capable of working.

How to Use This Book

This is not a book meant to be read once and placed on a shelf. It is a field guide you can return to at multiple stages of your journey: when you are considering nursing school, preparing for clinical rotations, entering the job market, transitioning specialties, or reassessing your long-term direction. Some readers will move through the book sequentially. Others will jump directly to the Day-in-the-Life sections to explore specific practice settings, then return later to the Hiring System or the decision-support tools. Both approaches are intentional. The goal is not speed; the goal is clarity. Each section is built to help you understand not only what nurses do, but how different roles feel, how hiring decisions are made, and how small career choices compound over time.

Throughout the book, you will also encounter reflection points, practical hiring strategies, and a specialty-focused version of the **SCRUB*fit*™** decision tools that help you evaluate which nursing environments align most closely with your personality, preferences, and long-term goals. These tools are not tests, and they are not predictions. They are mirrors designed to help you notice patterns in your own thinking so that your career decisions are intentional rather than accidental.

Why This Book Exists

Healthcare does not struggle to attract people who care. It struggles to place them in roles that fit who they are. When role, environment, expectations, and identity are misaligned, even talented and dedicated nurses can feel exhausted, discouraged, or uncertain about their future in the profession. When alignment is present, the same work can feel meaningful, sustainable, and deeply rewarding. The purpose of this book is to help you see those alignment factors earlier than most people do, before important career decisions become difficult to reverse.

Who This Book Is For (and Who It Isn't)

This book is for students considering nursing, newly licensed Registered Nurses entering the workforce, experienced nurses exploring specialty transitions, and healthcare professionals who want a clearer understanding of how nursing environments differ from one another. It is also for advisors, educators, recruiters, and healthcare leaders who want a realistic picture of how nurses experience the profession across settings.

This book is not designed to replace nursing school curriculum, licensure preparation, or clinical training resources. Instead, it complements those materials by focusing on lived-reality decision making: how the work unfolds across specialties, how hiring actually operates behind the scenes, and how to navigate your career deliberately as opportunities appear.

A Note on Alignment, Responsibility, and Choice

No single specialty represents nursing as a whole. Each environment carries its own pace, pressures, rewards, and long-term tradeoffs. Understanding those differences early gives you the ability to make decisions that support both your patients and your own sustainability in the profession. Alignment is not about finding a perfect job. It is about recognizing which environments allow you to contribute effectively while still remaining energized enough to continue the work over time. The more intentionally you approach these decisions, the more control you retain over the direction your nursing career ultimately takes.

Chapter 3

Who This Book Is For (and Who It Isn't)

This book is for students considering nursing, newly licensed Registered Nurses entering the workforce, experienced nurses exploring specialty transitions, and healthcare professionals who want a clearer understanding of how nursing environments differ from one another. It is also designed for advisors, educators, recruiters, and healthcare leaders who want a realistic, lived-reality view of how nurses experience the profession across settings.

Within these pages, we highlight a wide range of nursing environments through Day-in-the-Life dispatches, including Emergency, Operating Room, Medical-Surgical, Intensive Care, Cardiology, Surgical Services, Post-Acute Care, Outpatient Surgery, Gastroenterology, Plastics, Burn Care, Pediatrics, NICU, Occupational/Employee Health, Home Health, and additional outpatient and specialty practice settings such as physician-office nursing. These examples are intentionally diverse, but they represent only a portion of the nursing landscape. In reality, nursing includes hundreds of specialty pathways across hospitals, clinics, community programs, research environments, corporate health systems, public health agencies, education, telehealth, and emerging care models that continue to evolve each year. The purpose of highlighting selected specialties is not to limit your vision, but to provide a realistic cross-section of how dramatically daily nursing life can differ depending on environment, pace, autonomy, and patient population.

This book is not designed to replace nursing school curriculum, licensure preparation, or clinical training resources. Instead, it complements those materials by focusing on lived-reality decision making: how the work unfolds across specialties, how hiring actually operates behind the scenes, and how to navigate your career deliberately as opportunities appear.

Chapter 4

Meet the SCRUBfits™ — RN Edition

Registered nursing unfolds across environments that feel dramatically different from one another. The pace, emotional tone, patient population, and daily rhythm of the work change depending on where a nurse practices, and those differences often determine whether the role feels energizing or exhausting over time. The **SCRUB*fits*™** serve as alignment mirrors — helping you see how the same RN license can lead to very different lived experiences.

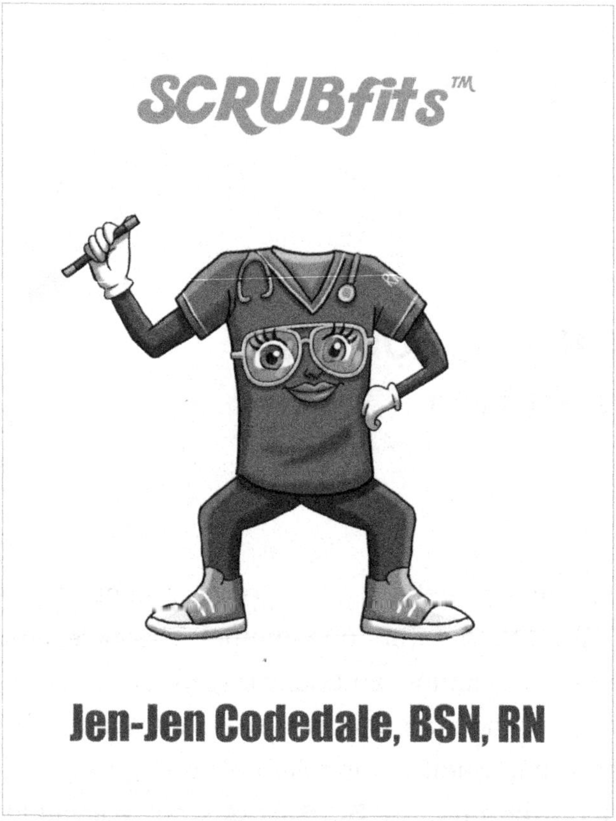

SCRUB*fit*™ Jen-Jen Codedale, RN, BSN — Emergency Department

Jen-Jen works in the Emergency Department, where the pace is unpredictable and urgency is constant. Patients arrive without warning, priorities shift within seconds, and rapid assessment drives nearly every decision. Nurses who feel focused rather than overwhelmed when the environment becomes fast and intense often recognize themselves in Jen-Jen's rhythm. Alignment here comes from comfort with uncertainty, quick decision-making, and the ability to reset emotionally between high-intensity encounters.

SCRUBfits™

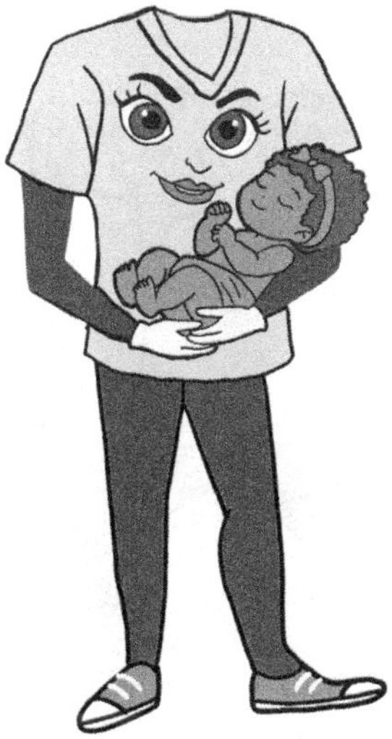

Hope Fulle, BSN, RN

SCRUB*fit*™ Hope Fulle, RN, BSN — Neonatal Intensive Care Unit (NICU)

Hope works in the Neonatal Intensive Care Unit, where precision, patience, and sustained vigilance shape each shift. The pace is not chaotic, but the responsibility is profound — small changes matter, quiet observation matters, and consistency across hours and days supports fragile patient progress. Nurses who thrive in highly detail-oriented environments where careful monitoring and long-term continuity guide the work often feel aligned with Hope's setting.

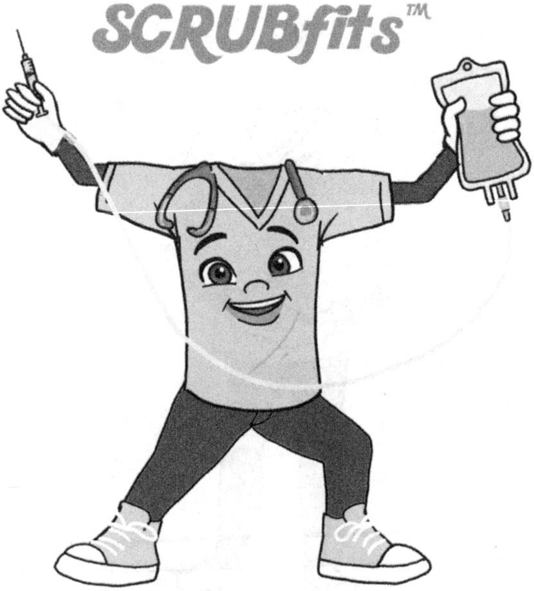

Suzette Soleil, RN

SCRUB*fit*™ Suzette Soleil, RN — Medical-Surgical Floor

Suzette practices on a medical-surgical floor, where steady movement defines the day. Multiple patients, frequent medication passes, interdisciplinary coordination, admissions, discharges, and family communication create a continuous operational rhythm. Nurses who appreciate structured variety — a predictable workflow combined with constantly changing patient needs — often find med-surg nursing both challenging and rewarding over time.

SCRUBfits™

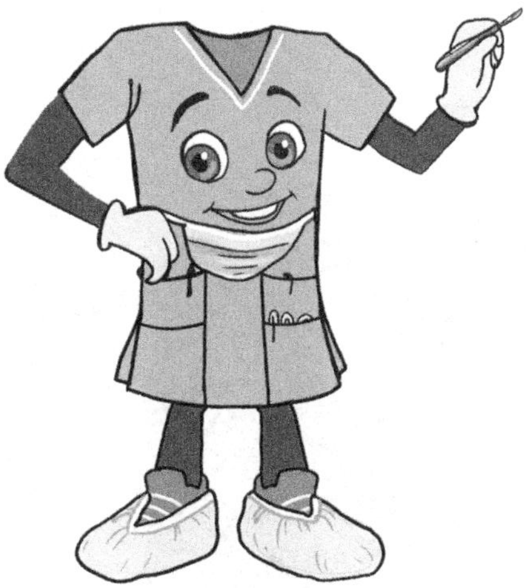

Brad Bovie, BSN, RN, CNOR

SCRUB*fit*™ Brad Bovie, RN, BSN, CNOR — Operating Room (OR) / Perioperative Nursing

Brad works in the Operating Room, where precision, preparation, and team choreography define the day. The pace can shift from calm setup to urgent response, but the work is always exacting — sterile technique, safety checks, instrument and sponge counts, documentation, and rapid coordination when a case changes unexpectedly. Nurses who feel energized by structure, technical accuracy, and anticipating the next step before it's needed often recognize themselves in Brad's rhythm. Alignment here comes from comfort with high standards, focused communication, and the satisfaction of cases that begin, progress, and reach clear completion points.

SCRUBfits™

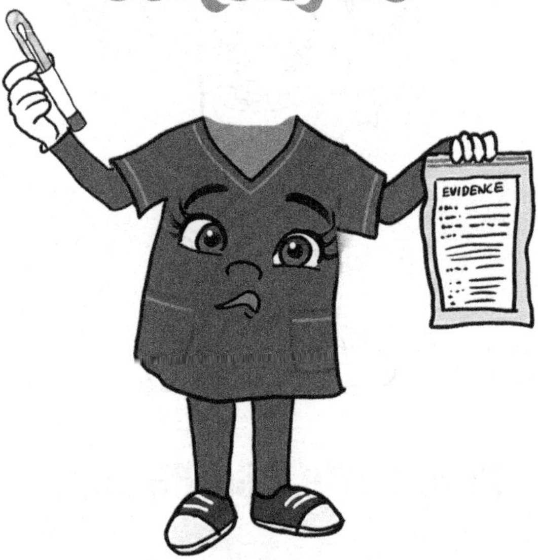

Justice Jules, RN, SANE-A

SCRUB*fit*™ Justice Jules, RN, SANE-A — Forensic Nursing / Emergency Response

Justice Jules works in forensic nursing environments, often connected to emergency departments and specialized advocacy programs. Her work requires clinical precision alongside documentation, patient protection, and legal-interface responsibilities. Nurses who feel strongly called to advocacy roles, where emotional steadiness and careful evidence handling are essential, often resonate with Justice's path.

SCRUBfits™

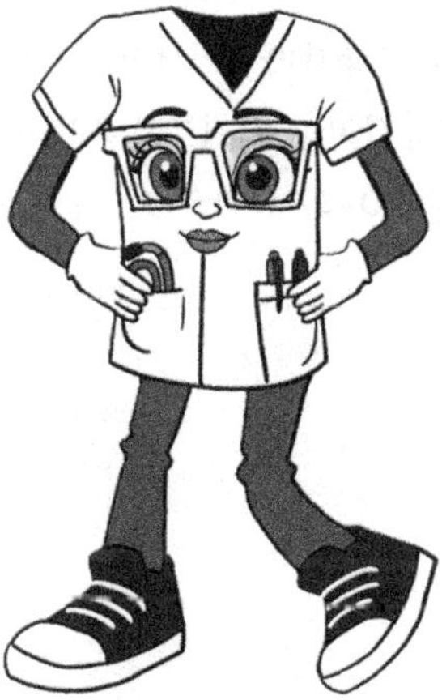

Anna Remedy,
DNP, FNP-BC

SCRUB*fit*™ Anna Remedy, DNP, FNP-BC, PMHNP — Advanced Practice Nursing

Anna represents the advanced-practice pathway available to Registered Nurses who pursue graduate education and specialty certification. As a Nurse Practitioner, she practices in primary care and behavioral health environments where diagnosing conditions, prescribing medications, and managing treatment plans become central responsibilities.

Her role illustrates how the RN pathway can expand into positions with broader clinical authority and independent decision-making depending on state scope-of-practice laws.

You may see yourself immediately in one of these environments, or you may recognize pieces of your preferences across several. That recognition is the purpose of the **SCRUB*fits*™**. Alignment is not only about becoming a nurse; it is about choosing the setting where the pace, responsibility level, and daily rhythm allow you to perform well and sustain your energy over time.

Chapter 5

A Note on Alignment, Responsibility, and Choice

A nursing license opens doors to an extraordinary range of career paths, but the availability of options does not automatically create clarity. Many nurses enter the profession with a general vision of helping others, only to discover that the daily experience of nursing varies dramatically depending on the environment in which the work takes place. Pace, acuity, patient interaction patterns, documentation demands, leadership culture, scheduling structure, and team dynamics can differ so widely across specialties that two nurses with identical credentials may experience completely different professional lives. Recognizing these differences early allows you to make career decisions with intention rather than reacting to whichever opportunity happens to appear first.

Alignment is not about finding a perfect job or eliminating challenge from the work. Nursing will always require resilience, responsibility, and the ability to perform under pressure. Alignment instead refers to the degree to which your personality, strengths, preferences, life circumstances, and long-term goals interact productively with the specific environment in which you practice. When alignment is present, the demands of the role often feel purposeful and manageable. When alignment is absent, even meaningful work can gradually feel exhausting or unsustainable over time. Understanding this distinction gives you the ability to make thoughtful adjustments—whether by changing units, pursuing additional training, transitioning specialties, or redefining your long-term career direction.

Responsibility and choice operate together throughout a nursing career. Healthcare systems, labor markets, staffing realities, and organizational cultures will always influence the opportunities available at any given moment, yet nurses still retain meaningful agency in how they prepare, which environments they pursue, how they evaluate offers, and when they decide to pivot. The purpose of this book is not to tell you which specialty to choose, but to provide a clearer lens through which to evaluate the options in front of you. The more intentionally you approach these decisions, the more likely you are to build a career that supports both your patients and your own long-term sustainability in the profession.

Chapter 6

The Toll Booth

The Emotional, Cognitive, and Lifestyle Cost of Registered Nursing

Every meaningful profession has a cost of entry that is not listed in the job description. In nursing, that cost is not measured only in tuition, clinical hours, or licensure exams. It is also measured in emotional exposure, cognitive demand, physical stamina, and the lifestyle adjustments required to sustain the work over time. Understanding this "toll" does not discourage the right people from entering nursing; instead, it prepares them to approach the profession with clarity and realistic expectations.

The emotional toll of nursing comes from repeated proximity to vulnerability. Nurses are present at moments patients and families often remember for the rest of their lives: unexpected diagnoses, sudden deteriorations, complex recoveries, and quiet conversations that happen when uncertainty fills the room. Even in outpatient or physician-office settings where acuity may be lower, the emotional dimension of care remains present through chronic disease management, patient education, and long-term relationship building. Over time, exposure to these moments can be deeply meaningful, but it can also require intentional strategies for emotional recovery so that compassion fatigue does not quietly accumulate.

The cognitive toll of nursing is equally significant. Nurses operate in environments where attention cannot drift and where small details can carry large consequences. Medication timing, assessment changes, subtle patient-condition shifts, equipment monitoring, and interdisciplinary communication require sustained mental focus across entire shifts. In high-acuity environments such as Emergency, ICU, or Burn units, the pace intensifies the cognitive load; in outpatient or procedural settings, precision and workflow timing create a different form of concentration demand. Regardless of the specialty, the work consistently requires rapid prioritization, situational awareness, and the ability to shift attention quickly while maintaining accuracy.

The physical toll is often underestimated before entering the profession. Long hours on one's feet, patient transfers, repositioning, equipment movement, and extended shift lengths—particularly 12-hour schedules—can challenge even individuals with strong physical endurance. Rotating schedules, night shifts, weekends, and holiday coverage further influence sleep patterns, recovery time, and long-term lifestyle balance. Some specialties offer more predictable scheduling, while others trade schedule stability for compensation differentials or higher-acuity clinical experiences. Recognizing these lifestyle variables early helps nurses make specialty decisions that align with their long-term health and personal priorities.

There is also a professional-responsibility toll that emerges as nurses gain experience. New graduates often focus primarily on learning clinical skills, but over time responsibilities expand to include mentoring new staff, coordinating care transitions, participating in committees, serving as charge nurses, or managing increasingly complex patient assignments. These added layers of responsibility are signs of professional growth, yet they also increase the decision-making load and time-management demands associated with the role.

None of these tolls exist to suggest that nursing is uniquely difficult compared to other professions. Rather, they illustrate that the realities of nursing extend beyond technical skill and academic preparation. When individuals understand the emotional, cognitive, and lifestyle costs of the profession before entering or transitioning specialties, they are better equipped to build routines, boundaries, and career strategies that sustain them long-term. Throughout the chapters that follow, you will see how the toll varies across nursing environments—sometimes intensifying, sometimes easing, but always present in different forms. Recognizing how these patterns interact with your own preferences, energy patterns, and long-term goals is one of the most important steps in building a nursing career that remains both meaningful and sustainable.

Chapter 7

Day In The Life — Emergency Department

Jen-Jen Codedale, RN, BSN, CEN — Shift Manager

Jordan Reyes, RN, BSN — Emergency Department Staff Nurse

Some readers may remember **Jen-Jen Codedale, RN, BSN** from *What Color Are Your Scrubs? (WCAYS).* At **Hopewell Hospital for Tomorrow**, she now serves as the shift manager at one of the system's freestanding emergency departments — facilities built for rapid stabilization, decisive clinical action, and tightly coordinated transfers to the main hospital when inpatient care is required. In this environment, the emergency department functions as both frontline treatment center and gateway, where clinical precision and operational timing determine how smoothly patients move to the next level of care. One of the nurses working under her leadership today is **Jordan Reyes, RN, BSN**, a steady emergency nurse known for calm bedside presence and rapid clinical instincts.

Jordan wakes before the alarm fully sounds, the room still dim with early-morning quiet. From the hallway, the steady sound of paws against hardwood announces that **Brutus**, the family's loyal German Shepherd, is already awake and waiting. Jordan stretches, swings out of bed, and heads to the kitchen while coffee brews and Brutus circles near the back door, ready for the first walk of the day. Breakfast is simple—eggs, toast, and a quick look at the shift schedule—followed by a short text from a spouse finishing a night shift at another hospital: "Quiet night. Sleep when you can tonight." These small exchanges are part of the rhythm of healthcare households, where schedules rarely align but understanding always does.

The drive to the freestanding ED takes about twenty minutes, long enough for Jordan to shift mentally into clinical mode. As the building comes into view, an EMS unit is already backing toward the ambulance bay, signaling that the department's pace has begun well before official shift start. Inside, the night team finishes charting while preparing handoff reports. At the center station stands Jen-Jen, scanning the tracking board and reviewing staffing coverage, incoming EMS alerts, and transfer timelines already in motion. She greets Jordan with a quick nod and a concise update: "Two potential cardiac transfers today, one stroke alert inbound, and imaging is tight this morning. You'll start in rooms four through six."

Within minutes, the shift is underway. Jordan begins with a chest-pain patient who arrived just before dawn, applying monitors, reviewing medications, and drawing labs while explaining each step in a calm, reassuring voice. Emergency nursing requires immediate clinical awareness paired with emotional steadiness; patients often arrive anxious, uncertain, or in pain, and the nurse becomes the first stable point in an unpredictable moment. As Jordan documents the initial assessment, the overhead radio call announces incoming EMS with stroke symptoms. The tempo changes instantly. Jen-Jen moves through the department clearing a high-acuity room, confirming imaging readiness, and notifying the main hospital's stroke team that a transfer may be imminent. By the time the stretcher reaches the bay, the operational path is already prepared.

The patient arrives, and the room fills with purposeful movement. Jordan assists with IV access and neurological assessments while the physician coordinates imaging orders. Just outside the room, Jen-Jen ensures transport availability and confirms the receiving facility's acceptance. In a freestanding ED, admission does not occur onsite; stabilization, decision-making, and transfer coordination are central parts of the workflow. Within an hour, the patient is stabilized, imaging is complete, and the transport team is preparing to move the patient to the main campus for definitive care. The sequence is fast, efficient, and carefully orchestrated—exactly how the system is designed to function.

The morning continues in waves. A pediatric respiratory case arrives requiring nebulizer treatments and observation. An elderly patient presents with confusion that may indicate infection or neurological change. Jordan moves steadily between rooms, balancing clinical priorities, documentation, and patient education while keeping reassessment intervals tight. Jen-Jen circulates continuously, adjusting staffing coverage as volumes rise, helping clear discharge bottlenecks, and coordinating pending transfers so no stabilized patient waits longer than necessary for transport.

By midday, the waiting area begins to fill. Two patients requiring inpatient monitoring are already in the transfer queue, with transport arrival times confirmed and receiving units notified at the main hospital. Jen-Jen reviews documentation completeness—labs, imaging, medication timelines, physician notes—ensuring that each patient's clinical story will transfer cleanly without missing information. Meanwhile, Jordan continues bedside care, administering medications, preparing transfer packets, and reassessing vital signs to confirm stability prior to departure. Their work intersects constantly: Jordan maintains direct clinical focus on the patient, while Jen-Jen manages the operational pathway that ensures the patient reaches the correct level of care without delay.

The early afternoon brings another surge. EMS radios ahead with a possible cardiac event. Jen-Jen immediately adjusts assignments, pulling additional coverage into Jordan's section and preparing the cardiac response equipment. When the patient arrives, Jordan initiates assessment and monitoring while Jen-Jen coordinates physician response and prepares the transfer call to the main hospital's cardiac unit. The teamwork is nearly silent but highly synchronized—each nurse operating within clearly understood roles that allow care to move quickly and safely.

A brief lull appears later in the afternoon, just long enough to restock trauma carts and check pending results. Jen-Jen walks the department floor, speaking briefly with each nurse, confirming staffing coverage for the evening surge, and reviewing transfer turnaround times. Leadership here is visible and mobile; rather than remaining in an office, the shift manager stays embedded in the clinical environment, reading flow patterns and adjusting resources in real time.

As evening approaches, patient volume rises again. Jordan manages multiple rooms, coordinating medications, discharge teaching, and reassessments while supporting a newly arrived nurse with orientation questions. Jen-Jen steps in periodically to help clear discharged patients, reassign rooms, and maintain safe staffing ratios as acuity fluctuates. Their collaboration reflects the balance required in emergency care: bedside clinical focus paired with system-level operational leadership, each supporting the other to keep the department functioning smoothly.

Shift change arrives quickly. Jordan gives bedside report, reviewing pending labs, medication schedules, and clinical concerns for each patient. Jen-Jen then briefs the incoming shift manager on department census, transfer timelines, staffing coverage, and anticipated overnight pressures. The goal is continuity. Even as individual shifts end, the system remains in motion, handing responsibility forward without interruption.

Outside, the evening air feels slower than the department left behind. Jordan walks to the car, shoulders gradually relaxing as the pace of the shift fades. At home, Brutus will be waiting at the door, ready to greet the end of another emergency-department day with steady enthusiasm. Tomorrow morning, the freestanding ED will already be moving again, and both Jordan and Jen-Jen will return—one anchoring the bedside, the other guiding the rhythm of the department—each role essential to the coordinated care that begins in this building and continues at the main hospital beyond it.

SCRUB*fits*™ Reflection — Jen-Jen Codedale, RN, BSN, CEN

"Freestanding emergency departments demand clinicians who can stabilize quickly, think clearly under pressure, and coordinate care across facilities without losing focus. If the pace of rapid assessments, constant reprioritizing, and tightly timed transfers felt energizing as you read this chapter, that reaction is meaningful. Emergency nursing is not only about clinical skill; it is about how well you function inside a fast-moving system where teamwork and timing shape patient outcomes minute by minute."

Chapter 8

Day In The Life — Operating Room

Melissa Grant, RN, CNOR wakes before dawn, the quiet of the house still unbroken except for the faint bubbling of the small aquarium on the kitchen counter. The soft glow of the tank light reflects across the room as she pours coffee and checks the surgery schedule on her phone—orthopedic block cases this morning, followed by a late-afternoon add-on procedure. Operating room nursing rewards preparation, and the day begins mentally long before entering the hospital.

Breakfast is quick—Greek yogurt, fruit, and a second cup of coffee poured into a travel mug. Her partner is still asleep after a late shift, so Melissa leaves a short handwritten note on the counter before heading out. The drive takes thirty minutes, enough time to review the surgical lineup mentally: total knee replacement, shoulder repair, and two outpatient procedures. In the OR, knowing the flow of the day before stepping inside makes everything smoother.

After changing into scrubs and securing her badge, **Melissa Grant, RN, CNOR** enters the surgical suite where the controlled rhythm of the operating department has already begun. Unlike many hospital units, the OR carries a quiet intensity—conversations are brief, movements purposeful, and preparation happens with meticulous precision. The circulating nurse role requires overseeing the entire environment: confirming patient identity, verifying procedure details, ensuring required implants and instruments are available, coordinating with anesthesia, and preparing documentation before the first incision ever occurs.

The first patient arrives from preoperative holding, anxious but calm. Melissa introduces herself, confirms identifiers, reviews allergies, and explains what will happen next. Even short conversations matter; for many patients, the circulating nurse becomes the last voice they remember before anesthesia begins. Once inside the room, equipment checks proceed systematically—monitors, positioning devices, sterile supplies, implant packaging, and surgical counts all verified before the team begins.

As the procedure starts, the operating room shifts into focused quiet. The surgeon works within the sterile field alongside the scrub nurse and surgical technologist, while Melissa moves just outside the field coordinating documentation, retrieving additional supplies, communicating with pathology or radiology when needed, and maintaining continuous awareness of the patient's overall status. OR nursing requires an unusual blend of stillness and readiness—long stretches of careful observation punctuated by moments where rapid coordination is essential.

Between cases, turnover happens quickly. Rooms are cleaned, new sterile trays opened, equipment repositioned, and the next patient prepared. Communication with the preoperative area ensures timing stays aligned; delays ripple across the entire surgical schedule if not managed carefully. By late morning, the orthopedic block is running smoothly, the team moving almost wordlessly through familiar routines built over months of working together.

Afternoon cases introduce variation. An unexpected instrument request requires a quick trip to sterile processing. A surgeon asks for an implant size adjustment, prompting coordination with supply staff. A family member calls requesting updates, and Melissa steps out briefly to provide reassurance. Circulating nurses serve as the operational bridge connecting surgical teams, patients, families, anesthesia staff, and perioperative leadership, often solving logistical challenges before others even notice them.

As the final procedure concludes, closing counts are confirmed, documentation finalized, and the patient transferred safely to recovery. The operating room gradually resets for the next day's schedule while staff begin wrapping up charting and supply checks. Unlike units where patient care continues indefinitely, the OR offers a defined closure to each case—a structured ending that many perioperative nurses find deeply satisfying.

Walking back through the locker room, Melissa changes out of scrubs and checks tomorrow's surgical assignments before heading to the parking garage. The drive home feels calm compared to the controlled intensity of the operating suite. At home, the aquarium light glows softly again, marking the return to a quieter pace. Dinner, a short walk, and a quick glance at the next day's schedule complete the routine, preparing for another morning where precision, preparation, and teamwork will once again define the work inside the operating room.

SCRUB*fit*™ Brad Bovie, RN, BSN, CNOR — Reflection

"When I read Melissa's day, what stands out immediately is the quiet discipline that defines operating room nursing. The environment isn't loud or chaotic most of the time — it's controlled, methodical, and intensely preparation-driven. Nurses who feel comfortable thinking three steps ahead, who gain satisfaction from precise coordination, sterile workflow, and team choreography, often feel deeply aligned in the OR. Much of the work happens before anything dramatic occurs: confirming implants, anticipating surgeon needs, maintaining counts, and ensuring every safety checkpoint is intact. If a nurse finds fulfillment in structured focus, technical accuracy, and the rhythm of cases that begin, progress, and reach clear completion points, the operating room can feel like a professional home. But for those who need constant patient interaction, unpredictable pacing, or continuous bedside connection, this same environment may feel too controlled or procedural. Alignment in perioperative nursing comes from recognizing whether precision and preparation energize you — or quietly drain you over time."

Chapter 9

Day In The Life — Medical-Surgical Unit

Angela Whitmore, RN, BSN wakes to the steady vibration of her phone alarm at **05:15**, the soft morning light just beginning to push through the bedroom curtains. Her cat, Milo, stretches across the edge of the bed as if protesting the early start. Angela reaches over, silences the alarm, and sits for a moment gathering the mental focus that med-surg nursing requires—today will involve multiple patients, multiple care plans, and constant prioritization.

In the kitchen, oatmeal warms on the stove while coffee brews. Her teenage son is already getting ready for school, and the two exchange quick morning updates about schedules before she packs a lunch—something learned after too many days relying on vending machines during busy shifts. By **06:00**, she's out the door, commuting twenty-five minutes to the hospital while listening to a short news podcast, a small routine that helps transition her mind into work mode.

After changing into scrubs and checking the assignment board, **Angela Whitmore, RN, BSN** receives report on five patients—typical for the medical-surgical floor. Each has a different diagnosis: post-operative recovery following abdominal surgery, uncontrolled diabetes requiring medication adjustment, pneumonia needing IV antibiotics, a fall patient under observation, and a patient preparing for discharge later that afternoon. Med-surg nursing is often described as the "backbone" of hospital care because it requires managing wide clinical variety simultaneously.

The morning begins with rapid assessments. Angela moves room to room checking vital signs, reviewing overnight changes, verifying medication schedules, and speaking briefly with each patient to understand immediate needs. One patient reports increased pain, another is anxious about an upcoming test, and a third needs assistance getting out of bed for the first time after surgery. Every interaction requires clinical attention combined with reassurance and clear explanation.

Medication administration follows, one of the most time-sensitive portions of the shift. Scanning systems confirm accuracy, and Angela double-checks dosages while answering questions from patients about new prescriptions. Between rooms, physicians round on the unit, and quick hallway conversations update treatment plans. Orders change, lab tests are scheduled, and discharge planning begins for patients nearing recovery.

Late morning brings the unpredictable rhythm typical of med-surg care. A patient's blood pressure drops slightly, prompting additional monitoring and a call to the provider. Another patient's family arrives with questions about recovery timelines. A physical therapist requests assistance ambulating a patient for the first time post-procedure. Angela balances each task while keeping a mental checklist of what must be completed next—charting updates, IV site checks, wound care, and education instructions for the patient preparing to go home.

Lunch rarely happens at a fixed time, but a coworker covers the floor for a short break, and Angela steps into the staff lounge long enough to eat the packed lunch from earlier. Conversations with fellow nurses are brief but supportive, sharing quick updates about patient conditions or helping one another anticipate the afternoon workload. Teamwork is essential; when the unit grows busy, nurses rely heavily on one another to maintain safe patient care.

Afternoon hours focus heavily on discharge coordination. Angela reviews medication instructions with one patient and family member, ensuring follow-up appointments are scheduled and warning signs clearly explained. Another patient requires additional teaching about insulin administration, and Angela spends extra time demonstrating technique and answering questions. Education is a central component of med-surg nursing—successful recovery often depends on what patients understand before leaving the hospital.

As evening approaches, charting becomes the final major task. Assessments, medication records, patient education notes, and provider communications must all be documented accurately. Before the night shift arrives, Angela performs final rounds—confirming comfort levels, ensuring call lights are within reach, and speaking briefly with each patient to address last-minute needs. These small end-of-shift check-ins often prevent overnight complications and help patients feel supported.

During handoff report, **Angela Whitmore, RN, BSN** reviews each case carefully with the incoming nurse: pending labs, medication changes, mobility concerns, and any behavioral or emotional needs worth noting. Clear communication ensures continuity of care, allowing the next shift to begin with confidence rather than uncertainty.

Driving home just after sunset, Angela reflects on the steady pace of the day. No single dramatic moment defined the shift, yet dozens of smaller interventions—pain control, medication adjustments, patient teaching, safe ambulation—collectively moved several patients closer to recovery. At home, Milo greets her at the door, and the evening routine settles into a quieter rhythm. Another day on the medical-surgical unit has ended, built not on a single emergency but on the consistent, coordinated care that keeps hospitals running and patients steadily healing.

SCRUB*fit*™ Suzette Soleil, RN — Reflection

"Angela's day is med-surg truth, start to finish: steady movement, constant prioritization, and five parallel storylines that you're holding in your head at the same time while the plan changes in real time. This is the kind of shift that doesn't usually come with one cinematic, 'big' moment, but it absolutely comes with impact — because the work is built out of dozens of small decisions that add up to recovery. When I read her morning, I can feel the operational rhythm: rapid assessments, med pass timing, quick

Chapter 10

Day In The Life — Intensive Care Unit

Daniel Cho, RN, BSN, CCRN wakes at **04:45**, well before sunrise, the early hour a familiar companion for ICU nurses working twelve-hour shifts. The apartment is quiet except for the low hum of the coffee machine programmed the night before. His Labrador, Atlas, lifts his head from the corner dog bed, tail thumping softly as Daniel walks into the kitchen. Morning routines are simple but intentional—coffee, oatmeal, a quick stretch, and a few minutes reviewing the patient census notes sent through the hospital's staffing app. ICU days demand mental readiness before the shift even begins.

The commute into the city takes thirty minutes. Traffic is light, and the gradual glow of sunrise reflects off the hospital's glass tower as Daniel pulls into employee parking. Inside the locker room, he changes into scrubs, clips his badge into place, and walks toward the intensive care unit where the overnight shift is already deep into early-morning assessments. The ICU carries a different energy than most hospital units—quieter in sound, heavier in responsibility.

Every patient requires continuous monitoring, and even small changes in vital signs can signal major clinical developments.

Report begins at the bedside. **Daniel Cho, RN, BSN, CCRN** receives two patients, a typical ICU ratio. The first is a post-cardiac-surgery patient requiring multiple IV drips, ventilator support, and frequent lab monitoring. The second is a severe pneumonia case on high-flow oxygen with fluctuating blood pressure overnight. Handoff includes medication titration ranges, lab trends, physician plans, family communication notes, and subtle observations from the night nurse—details that often matter as much as formal documentation.

The first hour moves quickly through detailed assessments. Daniel checks neurological status, ventilator settings, IV infusion rates, cardiac monitor rhythms, and fluid balance totals. ICU nursing requires constant prioritization while simultaneously maintaining precision; each patient has dozens of data points that must be observed, interpreted, and documented throughout the shift. When lab results return, medication adjustments may be required within minutes, and coordination with physicians and pharmacists becomes immediate.

Mid-morning brings a multidisciplinary bedside round. Physicians, respiratory therapists, pharmacists, and nursing staff gather briefly to review each patient's progress and adjust treatment plans. Daniel provides updates on overnight stability, urine output changes, sedation response, and family concerns. ICU nurses serve as the continuous observers at the bedside, often noticing early clinical trends before anyone else, making their input central to care planning discussions.

Family members begin arriving later in the morning, and communication shifts tone. For relatives, the ICU environment can feel overwhelming—monitors, alarms, and unfamiliar equipment creating visible anxiety. Daniel explains what each device does, clarifies treatment steps, and answers questions with calm, measured pacing. These conversations require emotional steadiness; families often look to the bedside nurse for reassurance even during uncertain clinical situations.

The afternoon demands sustained attention. A medication titration is adjusted based on blood pressure response, respiratory therapy performs ventilator setting changes, and lab draws are repeated to evaluate electrolyte levels. ICU work often alternates between long periods of focused monitoring and brief moments where rapid intervention is required. When an alarm signals a rhythm change on the cardiac monitor, Daniel responds immediately, assessing the patient and coordinating quickly with the care team before stability returns.

Documentation continues throughout the day, detailed and time-sensitive. Unlike other units where charting may occur in blocks, ICU charting often happens in real time because patient conditions can change minute by minute. Intake and output calculations, medication titration logs, neurological assessments, and ventilator responses all require precise recording to maintain continuity across shifts.

As evening approaches, the unit quiets slightly, though never completely. Daniel prepares end-of-shift reports, reviewing lab trends, medication adjustments, and any subtle clinical changes the incoming nurse should monitor closely. ICU handoffs are thorough; the accuracy of this transfer directly affects patient safety over the next twelve hours.

Walking to the parking garage after the shift, the outside air feels noticeably lighter than the intensity of the unit left behind. The drive home becomes a gradual mental decompression—thinking briefly about the patients who stabilized, hoping for continued improvement overnight, then intentionally shifting attention back to personal life. Atlas greets him enthusiastically at the door, an immediate reminder that the hospital world has paused for now. Dinner, a short walk with the dog, and a quiet evening allow the day's intensity to settle, preparing for another shift where vigilance, precision, and calm decision-making will again define the work inside the intensive care unit.

Chapter 11

Day In The Life — Cardiology Unit

Priya Natarajan, RN, BSN wakes at **05:30** to the soft chime of her phone alarm, the early morning still quiet outside the apartment windows. Her husband is already in the kitchen preparing coffee, and the smell reaches the bedroom just as she swings her feet onto the floor. Their small terrier, Rocco, trots excitedly down the hallway, ready for his short morning walk. Priya pulls on a sweatshirt, clips the leash, and steps outside into the cool morning air, using the ten-minute walk around the block as a gentle transition into the day ahead.

Back home, breakfast is quick—toast, yogurt, and coffee poured into a travel mug while she reviews the patient assignment notification sent through the hospital scheduling system. Cardiology shifts often involve a mix of telemetry monitoring, medication titration, and post-procedure recovery, and knowing the general census before arriving helps her mentally organize priorities. By **06:15**, she is in the car for the twenty-minute commute, listening to music while traffic gradually thickens near the hospital campus.

After changing into scrubs and checking the telemetry board, **Priya Natarajan, RN, BSN** receives report on four cardiac patients. One is recovering from a cardiac catheterization procedure, another is being monitored for arrhythmia episodes, a third is adjusting to new heart-failure medications, and the fourth is preparing for a stress test later that day. Cardiology nursing blends continuous monitoring with patient education, requiring both technical awareness and clear communication.

Morning rounds begin with rhythm checks and full assessments. Priya reviews telemetry strips, verifying heart rhythm stability while checking vital signs, medication schedules, and fluid restrictions. Cardiac patients often require frequent medication adjustments, and she coordinates closely with physicians and pharmacists to ensure timing aligns with lab results and response patterns. One patient expresses anxiety about a new diagnosis, and Priya takes several minutes to explain the purpose of each medication, using diagrams to make the treatment plan easier to understand.

Late morning brings procedural follow-up. A patient returning from the catheterization lab requires groin-site monitoring, vital sign checks, and strict positioning instructions to prevent complications. Priya explains movement restrictions, checks for bleeding, and updates documentation while coordinating with the physician regarding post-procedure observations. Nearby, a telemetry alarm signals a rhythm change in another room. She quickly verifies whether the reading reflects patient movement or a genuine arrhythmia, confirming stability before resetting the monitor.

The unit's pace remains steady throughout the afternoon. Family members arrive with questions about lifestyle changes, dietary recommendations, and activity restrictions following discharge. Education plays a central role in cardiology nursing—patients often leave with medication adjustments and long-term management plans that depend heavily on understanding daily habits. Priya reviews sodium restrictions, medication timing, and follow-up appointments with one patient preparing to go home, ensuring written instructions match the physician's final orders.

Collaboration defines the workflow. Physical therapists assess mobility tolerance, dietitians review nutrition plans, and physicians conduct mid-afternoon rounds updating treatment strategies. Nurses serve as the central coordinators connecting each component of the patient's care plan, ensuring communication flows accurately between departments. Between tasks, Priya documents rhythm trends, medication responses, and patient teaching sessions, keeping records current for the evening shift.

As handoff approaches, she completes final telemetry reviews and reassesses each patient, confirming stability and comfort levels. During report, **Priya Natarajan, RN, BSN** summarizes rhythm observations, pending labs, medication adjustments, and discharge planning notes for the incoming nurse, ensuring no critical detail is overlooked.

Driving home at sunset, the intensity of the monitoring environment gradually fades. Cardiology nursing rarely involves the dramatic pace of the emergency department, yet the responsibility of watching for subtle rhythm changes carries its own form of constant vigilance. At home, Rocco greets her at the door, and the evening settles into a calmer rhythm—dinner, conversation, and a few quiet moments before preparing for another day helping patients navigate the delicate balance of cardiac recovery and long-term heart health.

Chapter 12

Day In The Life — Surgical Services

Anthony Delgado, RN, BSN wakes at **05:00**, the early hour familiar to anyone working surgical schedules that begin long before most of the city is awake. The house is quiet except for the faint clinking of his cat, Pepper, moving around the kitchen looking for breakfast. Anthony feeds the cat, pours coffee into a travel mug, and reviews the day's surgical assignment on his phone—several general surgery cases followed by an afternoon add-on procedure that was scheduled late the previous evening.

Breakfast is quick—two eggs, toast, and a short conversation with his spouse before heading out the door. The twenty-five-minute commute gives him time to mentally review the surgical flow: patient preparation, coordination with anesthesia, room readiness, and postoperative transfers. Surgical services nursing depends heavily on preparation, and the smoother the setup, the more efficiently the entire day runs.

After arriving at the hospital and changing into scrubs, **Anthony Delgado, RN, BSN** checks the operating schedule posted in the surgical services coordination area. Unlike the circulating nurse role that stays inside a single operating room, surgical services nurses often move between preoperative preparation, intraoperative coordination, and postoperative transitions, helping maintain continuity across the surgical process. The first patient of the day is already in the preoperative holding area, reviewing consent forms and waiting for final clearance.

Anthony begins with a calm introduction, confirming identity bands, allergies, and surgical details while answering a few last-minute patient questions. For many individuals, this stage carries the highest anxiety of the entire experience, and a few reassuring explanations about the process can make a significant difference. Once anesthesia staff arrive, he coordinates timing for transport to the operating suite while ensuring all required documentation is complete.

The morning progresses in a steady rhythm—preoperative preparations, room turnover coordination, equipment checks, and postoperative transfer communication with recovery staff. Surgical services nursing often functions as the connective tissue between departments, ensuring that patients move safely and efficiently through each phase of care. When a scheduled case runs longer than expected, Anthony communicates with pre-op staff to adjust timing, preventing unnecessary waiting for the next patient.

Midday brings a brief pause between procedures, just long enough to restock supplies and confirm readiness for the afternoon schedule. An add-on case requires rapid coordination—contacting sterile processing, confirming surgeon availability, and ensuring anesthesia coverage aligns with the new timeline. These operational adjustments happen frequently in surgical environments, and experienced nurses learn to adapt quickly without disrupting patient flow.

Throughout the afternoon, Anthony assists with postoperative transitions, receiving patients from the operating room and ensuring smooth handoff to recovery nurses. Vital signs are confirmed, documentation reviewed, and any special post-procedure instructions communicated clearly. These transitions are short but critical moments where accurate information prevents complications later in recovery.

As the final case concludes, the surgical area gradually quiets. Equipment is secured, documentation completed, and the next day's preliminary schedule reviewed. Surgical services rarely ends precisely at shift time—unexpected cases occasionally extend the day—but today's schedule finishes close to plan.

Walking back to the parking lot, Anthony reflects briefly on how many coordinated steps occurred behind the scenes for each patient who moved through surgery that day. Most patients remember only a few moments of the process, yet dozens of professionals contributed to each safe procedure. At home, Pepper waits near the door, dinner already on the evening schedule, and the day settles into a slower pace before the next early morning shift begins again.

SCRUB*fit*™ Brad Bovie, RN, BSN, CNOR — Reflection

"Anthony's day highlights something many people don't immediately see about perioperative nursing: surgery is not

only what happens inside the operating room; it's the orchestration that happens before and after the incision that keeps the entire system functioning safely. What stands out here is the operational mindset — anticipating schedule shifts, coordinating pre-op readiness, managing turnovers, and ensuring that every transition point is clean, clear, and documented. Nurses who feel energized by systems thinking, who naturally watch the flow of the day rather than only the task in front of them, often find strong alignment in surgical services roles. This work rewards preparation, communication precision, and the ability to adjust calmly when schedules change or add-on cases appear. For nurses who prefer long-term bedside relationships, the rapid transitions between patients may feel less personally connected; however, for those who appreciate the choreography of surgical care — where each well-timed handoff directly contributes to patient safety — the environment can feel deeply satisfying. Anthony's shift shows that perioperative nursing is as much about managing the pathway as it is about managing the procedure, and for nurses who enjoy keeping complex clinical operations moving smoothly, that responsibility becomes a powerful source of professional alignment."

Chapter 13

Day In The Life — Outpatient Surgery

Kevin Patel, RN, BSN wakes at **05:15**, the quiet of the morning broken only by the gentle alarm tone on his phone. His wife is already in the kitchen preparing coffee, and their two young children are still asleep upstairs, giving him a few calm minutes before the day begins. Kevin pours coffee into a travel mug, grabs a quick breakfast—banana, yogurt, and toast—and checks the outpatient surgery center's case lineup through the scheduling app. Today includes several orthopedic procedures, two endoscopic cases, and a late-afternoon plastic surgery add-on.

After a short twenty-minute commute, he parks near the ambulatory surgery center entrance and changes into scrubs. **Kevin Patel, RN, BSN** begins the morning by reviewing patient charts, verifying consent forms, allergies, and procedure requirements before the first patients arrive. Outpatient surgery nursing moves quickly but predictably—patients arrive, undergo procedures, recover briefly, and return home the same day, requiring efficient coordination across every stage of care.

The first patient check-in begins shortly after **06:30**. Kevin introduces himself, confirms identification bands, reviews medical history, and explains the sequence of events leading up to the procedure. Many patients feel nervous despite the routine nature of outpatient surgeries, and clear explanations often ease anxiety. Once preoperative preparation is complete, he coordinates transport to the procedure room while ensuring anesthesia staff have completed their evaluations.

Between cases, Kevin assists with room turnover preparation, equipment checks, and supply restocking to keep the surgical schedule running smoothly. Unlike inpatient operating rooms where patients may remain hospitalized afterward, outpatient settings require careful discharge preparation from the beginning—patients must meet recovery criteria, understand medication instructions, and have transportation arranged before leaving.

Late morning brings a steady rhythm of patient flow. One patient recovers quickly and is ready for discharge education within an hour, while another requires extended observation due to mild postoperative nausea. Kevin monitors vital signs, administers medications as ordered, and communicates with anesthesia providers to ensure each patient meets safety standards before release. Family members waiting in the recovery area often have questions about recovery timelines, activity restrictions, and pain management, and he takes time to review written instructions carefully.

The afternoon schedule continues with a mix of procedures, each requiring preoperative verification, intraoperative coordination, and postoperative monitoring. Outpatient surgery nursing demands constant attention to detail because patients leave the facility soon after procedures; discharge instructions must be accurate and clearly understood. Kevin reviews medication timing, wound care instructions, and follow-up appointment details with each patient before final sign-off.

As the final case concludes, documentation is completed and supply inventories are checked for the next day's procedures. Compared to inpatient hospital settings, the outpatient surgery center quiets quickly once the last patient is discharged, bringing a defined close to the workday.

Driving home in late afternoon traffic, Kevin reflects on the efficiency of outpatient surgical care—patients arriving early in the day and returning home safely just hours later. At home, his children greet him excitedly at the door, and the evening transitions into family time, homework help, and dinner preparation before the next day's surgical schedule begins again.

SCRUB*fit*™ Brad Bovie, RN, BSN, CNOR — Reflection

"Kevin's day illustrates the procedural rhythm that defines ambulatory surgery nursing — efficient, tightly coordinated, and highly preparation-driven. Unlike inpatient surgical environments where recovery may unfold over days, outpatient settings compress the entire surgical journey into a matter of hours, which means precision in education, verification, and discharge readiness becomes just as critical as the procedure itself. Nurses who feel energized by workflow efficiency,

structured patient flow, and the satisfaction of seeing patients safely arrive, undergo treatment, and return home the same day often find strong alignment in this environment. The pace is steady rather than chaotic, but the margin for communication errors is small because patients leave quickly after care. For nurses who enjoy predictable scheduling, clear beginning-to-end case cycles, and a strong operational focus, ambulatory surgical nursing can feel deeply sustainable over the long term. Kevin's shift demonstrates that surgical nursing is not defined only by the operating room itself — it is defined by the coordinated system that surrounds each procedure, where preparation, verification, and patient education quietly determine outcomes."

Chapter 14

Day In The Life — Post-Acute Care Unit

Linda Martinez, RN, BSN wakes at **06:00**, the soft morning light already filling the bedroom. Unlike hospital night shifts she worked earlier in her career, her current post-acute care schedule follows a more predictable daytime rhythm, something she intentionally chose after years in high-acuity settings. In the kitchen, her husband is preparing coffee while their small rescue dog, Bella, waits patiently near the door for her morning walk. Linda clips on the leash, and the short walk around the neighborhood becomes a quiet moment to ease into the day.

Breakfast is simple—fruit, toast, and coffee—before she gathers her badge, lunch bag, and car keys. The drive to the rehabilitation hospital takes about fifteen minutes, giving her just enough time to review the day's expected admissions and discharges through the facility's staff portal. Post-acute care nursing centers heavily on recovery planning, patient education, and interdisciplinary coordination, and knowing which patients are arriving or leaving helps frame the day's priorities.

After clocking in, **Linda Martinez, RN, BSN** receives report on her patient assignment—individuals recovering from surgeries, strokes, orthopedic procedures, and extended hospital stays who now require rehabilitation before returning home. Each patient is medically stable but still needs nursing oversight, medication management, and coordination with therapy teams. The morning begins with assessments, medication passes, and conversations with patients about therapy schedules planned for later in the day.

One patient recovering from hip surgery needs assistance preparing for physical therapy, while another stroke-recovery patient requires monitoring for blood pressure changes during activity sessions. Linda collaborates closely with physical and occupational therapists, ensuring medications are timed appropriately so patients can participate fully in rehabilitation. In post-acute care, nursing supports the recovery process not only through clinical care but also by helping patients regain confidence in their daily abilities.

Late morning brings discharge planning discussions. A patient preparing to return home meets with family members, and Linda reviews medication schedules, wound care instructions, and follow-up appointment requirements. Education plays a central role in this setting; successful recovery often depends on what patients understand before leaving the facility. She answers questions, clarifies mobility precautions, and ensures written instructions match the physician's orders.

Afternoon hours move at a steady but purposeful pace. New admissions arrive from acute-care hospitals, requiring intake assessments, medication reconciliation, and orientation to the rehabilitation program. Linda checks that therapy teams have the necessary information to begin evaluations, coordinating across departments to ensure care transitions remain smooth. Communication is constant—updates to physicians, therapy teams, case managers, and families all happen throughout the shift.

As the day winds down, documentation becomes the final priority—therapy participation notes, medication updates, patient education records, and discharge summaries must all be entered before the evening shift begins. During handoff, **Linda Martinez, RN, BSN** reviews patient progress, scheduled therapies, and any concerns requiring overnight monitoring.

Driving home in the early evening, Linda reflects on the different pace of post-acute nursing compared to her earlier hospital roles. While emergencies are less frequent, the satisfaction of watching patients regain strength and independence brings its own sense of fulfillment. At home, Bella greets her at the door, dinner preparations begin, and the evening settles into a calm routine, marking the end of another day helping patients move steadily toward recovery.

SCRUB*fit*™ Brad Bovie, RN, BSN, CNOR — Reflection

"Linda's day reflects a side of nursing that many clinicians discover later in their careers: the shift from crisis-driven care to recovery-centered care. What stands out is the intentional pace — still structured, still clinically focused, but designed around rebuilding strength rather than stabilizing emergencies. Nurses who find satisfaction in watching measurable progress over days or weeks, who enjoy patient education, discharge planning, and interdisciplinary coordination with therapy teams, often feel strongly aligned in post-acute and rehabilitation settings. This environment rewards patience, consistency, and clear communication more than rapid-response intensity. For nurses who thrive on adrenaline or moment-to-moment unpredictability, the rhythm may feel slower than preferred, but for those who value continuity, patient relationships, and the visible arc of recovery, this setting can feel deeply meaningful. Linda's experience shows that nursing alignment is not only about skill level or specialty—it is about choosing the pace, responsibility pattern, and emotional rhythm that allow you to sustain your energy over the long term."

Chapter 15

Day In The Life — Gastroenterology Unit

Rachel Kim, RN, BSN wakes at **05:40**, the soft vibration of her smartwatch alarm gently pulling her from sleep. Her apartment is quiet except for the rhythmic clicking of the ceiling fan, and her tabby cat, Oliver, immediately stretches across the bed as if requesting breakfast. Rachel smiles, feeds him, and heads into the kitchen where coffee brews while she prepares a quick breakfast—oatmeal topped with fruit and a boiled egg for extra protein. Gastroenterology nursing days often involve a steady procedural flow, and starting the morning organized helps everything run more smoothly.

By **06:15**, she is in her car for the twenty-minute drive to the hospital's endoscopy center, listening to a short podcast while mentally reviewing the day's schedule—screening colonoscopies, diagnostic upper endoscopies, and one therapeutic procedure scheduled for late morning. After changing into scrubs and checking the assignment board, **Rachel Kim, RN, BSN** begins preparing pre-procedure rooms, ensuring monitoring equipment is functioning and documentation packets are ready.

The first patient arrives shortly after **07:00**, slightly anxious about the upcoming procedure. Rachel introduces herself, verifies identity and allergies, reviews medication history, and explains what to expect before, during, and after the procedure. Patient education plays a significant role in gastroenterology nursing; many individuals arrive uncertain about preparation steps or recovery expectations, and clear communication helps reduce stress before sedation begins.

As procedures begin, Rachel assists with pre-procedure preparation, IV placement, and monitoring coordination while working closely with physicians, anesthesia providers, and technicians. Between cases, rooms are cleaned and reset quickly, maintaining the procedural flow that allows multiple patients to receive care efficiently throughout the day. Timing is important—delays in preparation can cascade across the entire schedule.

Late morning brings a slightly more complex therapeutic procedure requiring additional equipment preparation and closer post-procedure observation. Rachel coordinates with recovery-area staff to ensure monitoring plans are in place before the patient leaves the procedure room. In gastroenterology settings, recovery education is critical because most patients return home the same day. She reviews dietary instructions, medication guidelines, and warning signs patients should monitor once discharged.

Afternoon hours move steadily through the remaining schedule. Some patients recover quickly and are discharged within an hour, while others require additional monitoring due to sedation effects or minor complications. Rachel communicates frequently with family members waiting in the designated area, providing updates that help reduce anxiety during the short but often stressful waiting period.

Documentation continues between patient transitions—procedure notes, medication administration records, and discharge education confirmations must all be completed accurately before patients leave the facility. As the final cases wrap up, supplies are restocked, equipment cleaned, and the next day's preliminary case list reviewed.

Driving home in the early evening, Rachel reflects on the structured pace of procedural nursing compared to the unpredictability of acute-care hospital units she worked earlier in her career. At home, Oliver greets her at the door, circling her legs while she sets down her bag. Dinner preparation begins, the apartment quiet once again, and the day closes with the satisfaction of knowing dozens of patients received preventive and diagnostic care that may significantly influence their long-term health outcomes.

Chapter 16

Day In The Life — Plastic Surgery

Elena Vasquez, RN, BSN wakes at **05:30**, the early morning quiet broken only by the faint rustle of the palm trees outside her apartment balcony. Her small parakeet, Azul, chirps softly from his cage as she moves through the kitchen preparing coffee and a light breakfast—avocado toast and fruit. Plastic surgery nursing requires both procedural efficiency and patient-centered communication, and Elena values starting the day calm and organized before the schedule begins.

By **06:15**, she is driving to the outpatient surgical center where she works, reviewing the case list mentally—reconstructive procedures in the morning followed by cosmetic outpatient surgeries in the afternoon. After changing into scrubs, **Elena Vasquez, RN, BSN** checks the patient flow board, confirming arrival times, recovery room assignments, and discharge instructions prepared in advance. Plastic surgery nursing often involves shorter procedures but requires meticulous attention to postoperative care details because patients return home the same day.

The first patient arrives early, undergoing reconstructive surgery following a previous injury. Elena introduces herself, reviews consent forms, verifies allergies, and explains the recovery timeline carefully, knowing many patients feel both hopeful and anxious about surgical outcomes. Clear communication before procedures helps patients understand expectations and reduces postoperative confusion.

Once the surgical team begins, Elena coordinates preoperative preparation and recovery planning, ensuring supplies, dressings, and postoperative medications are ready before the patient enters recovery. Between cases, rooms are reset quickly while she checks in with family members waiting in designated areas, providing updates and estimated timelines.

Late morning transitions into cosmetic procedures requiring detailed postoperative education. Patients receiving elective treatments often have extensive questions about swelling, activity restrictions, medication use, and follow-up appointments. Elena reviews written discharge instructions thoroughly, demonstrating dressing changes and ensuring patients understand how to recognize warning signs that require medical attention.

The afternoon moves quickly as outpatient procedures continue. Coordination with anesthesia providers, surgeons, and recovery staff keeps patient flow smooth, while Elena monitors recovery patients closely for pain control and stable vital signs. Documentation follows each patient transition—procedure notes, medication administration records, and discharge confirmations entered before the next case begins.

As the final patient is discharged, the center gradually quiets. Elena restocks recovery supplies, checks the following day's schedule, and completes final charting before changing out of scrubs. Walking to the parking lot, she reflects on the balance of reconstructive and cosmetic work within plastic surgery nursing—some patients recovering from trauma or medical conditions, others pursuing elective procedures that significantly affect self-confidence and quality of life.

At home, Azul greets her with energetic chirps, and the evening settles into a relaxed routine—dinner, a short workout, and a call to family before preparing for another day where precision, patient education, and coordinated teamwork define the rhythm of plastic surgery nursing.

Chapter 17

Day In The Life — Burn Unit

Marcus Hill, RN, BSN, CCRN wakes at **04:50**, the alarm tone quiet but persistent. The apartment is still dark, the city only beginning to stir outside the window. His German shepherd, Titan, lifts his head from the corner bed, already sensing the start of the day. Marcus pours coffee, prepares a quick breakfast—eggs and toast—and spends a few minutes stretching, knowing the physical demands of burn-unit nursing require stamina as much as clinical skill.

The drive to the regional burn center takes about thirty minutes. As he approaches the hospital campus, the distinctive trauma entrance comes into view, a reminder that many burn patients arrive under urgent circumstances. After changing into scrubs, **Marcus Hill, RN, BSN, CCRN** enters the burn intensive care unit, where the overnight shift is completing assessments. Burn nursing requires a highly specialized skill set—pain management, wound care, infection prevention, fluid balance monitoring, and emotional support for patients facing long recovery journeys.

During report, Marcus receives two high-acuity patients. One is recovering from a house fire injury requiring extensive wound dressings and fluid monitoring; the second is a workplace injury patient undergoing staged surgical reconstruction. The handoff includes medication infusions, dressing change schedules, lab trends, and family communication notes. Burn care demands continuity, and even small details passed between shifts can significantly affect patient outcomes.

Morning assessments begin immediately. Marcus reviews vital signs, evaluates wound sites, checks IV infusions, and collaborates with physicians and wound-care specialists to plan dressing changes scheduled later in the morning. Dressing procedures can be lengthy and painful, requiring coordinated pain management strategies involving both medications and emotional support. He explains each step carefully to the patient before beginning, ensuring comfort measures are in place.

Late morning brings multidisciplinary rounds involving surgeons, nurses, therapists, dietitians, and social workers. Burn recovery requires coordinated care across many specialties—nutrition plans to support healing, physical therapy to maintain mobility, and psychological support to help patients cope with trauma. Marcus contributes bedside observations, noting subtle changes in wound appearance and patient tolerance to treatment.

Throughout the afternoon, he monitors fluid balance, adjusts dressings as ordered, and assists therapists working with patients beginning early mobility exercises. Conversations with family members are often emotional; burn injuries frequently involve long hospital stays and uncertain recovery timelines. Marcus answers questions patiently, helping families understand the treatment process while providing reassurance during difficult moments.

Documentation is detailed and continuous, reflecting wound assessments, medication responses, fluid intake and output, and patient progress notes. Burn nursing requires precision because infection prevention and treatment adjustments depend heavily on accurate charting. As evening approaches, Marcus prepares for shift handoff, reviewing each patient's wound-care schedule, medication plans, and overnight monitoring needs with the incoming nurse.

Leaving the hospital after the shift, the intensity of the burn unit lingers briefly in his thoughts. The drive home becomes a quiet decompression period, the evening traffic moving steadily while the day's pace gradually slows. Titan greets him enthusiastically at the door, a familiar routine that signals the transition from hospital intensity to home life. Dinner, a short walk, and a few moments of rest close the day, preparing for another shift dedicated to some of the most complex and resilient patients in acute-care nursing.

Chapter 18

Day In The Life — Pediatrics

Hannah Brooks, RN, BSN, CPN wakes at **05:20**, the soft glow of the baby monitor lighting the nightstand as her toddler shifts quietly in the next room. She listens for a moment, hears steady breathing, and slips out of bed to start the morning routine. In the kitchen, coffee brews while her orange tabby cat, Sunny, circles near the food bowl. Hannah prepares oatmeal, packs a small lunch, and checks the pediatric unit census on her phone—two respiratory cases, one post-appendectomy admission, and several children preparing for discharge later today.

Her husband begins getting their toddler ready for daycare while Hannah finishes breakfast and gathers her bag. By **06:10**, she is on the road for the twenty-minute commute to the children's hospital, using the drive to mentally prepare for the emotional balance pediatric nursing requires—clinical precision combined with communication tailored both to children and their families.

After changing into scrubs decorated with colorful pediatric-themed patterns, **Hannah Brooks, RN, BSN, CPN** receives bedside report on four patients. Pediatric assignments are structured differently than adult units, often factoring in developmental needs, family presence, and emotional support requirements alongside medical conditions. The first patient is a six-year-old admitted overnight for asthma exacerbation, the second a toddler recovering from surgery, and the remaining two children are being monitored for dehydration following viral illness.

Morning assessments begin gently. Hannah kneels beside the first patient rather than standing over the bed, speaking at eye level to explain the blood pressure cuff and stethoscope before beginning the exam. Pediatric nursing requires creativity and patience; small steps—letting a child hold the thermometer first or counting together during an injection—often make procedures far less stressful. Parents watch closely, and clear explanations help reassure them as much as the children.

Mid-morning brings medication administration, respiratory treatments, and coordination with pediatricians during rounds. One young patient requires breathing treatments every few hours, and Hannah works with respiratory therapy to ensure timing aligns with medication schedules. Another child is preparing for discharge, and she spends extra time teaching the parents medication dosing instructions, emphasizing safety and follow-up care.

Throughout the day, the pediatric unit carries a different emotional atmosphere than adult care settings. Laughter from playrooms mixes with the beeping of monitors, and staff members often keep small toys or stickers in their pockets to comfort anxious children during procedures. Teamwork is constant—child life specialists assist during blood draws, physicians round frequently, and nurses communicate closely with families to ensure every step of care is clearly understood.

Afternoon hours focus on reassessments, discharge preparation, and comforting a newly admitted patient frightened by the unfamiliar hospital environment. Hannah sits briefly with the child and parent, explaining what will happen next in simple terms while helping the child choose a stuffed animal from the comfort cart. Moments like these, though small, shape how families remember their hospital experience.

As the evening shift arrives, Hannah completes handoff report, detailing medication schedules, behavioral preferences, parental concerns, and any clinical changes requiring close monitoring overnight. Pediatric reporting often includes developmental or emotional details—favorite distractions, communication preferences, or calming techniques—that help the next nurse connect quickly with the child.

Driving home at sunset, she reflects on the day's mixture of technical care and emotional reassurance. Pediatric nursing demands both, often within the same minute. At home, her toddler runs to the door for a hug, Sunny weaving between their feet, and the evening transitions into dinner, bath time, and bedtime stories before the cycle begins again the next morning.

Chapter 19

Day In The Life — Neonatal Intensive Care Unit (NICU)

Lauren Mitchell, RN, BSN, RNC-NIC wakes at **04:40**, the early hour softened by the quiet hum of the humidifier near the bedroom window. Her husband is still asleep, and the house remains still except for the gentle scratching of their rescue cat, Willow, stretching near the hallway. Lauren moves quietly into the kitchen, pours coffee, and prepares a small breakfast—granola, yogurt, and fruit—while reviewing the NICU assignment notification on her phone. Neonatal nursing requires precision and emotional steadiness, and she prefers arriving mentally prepared for the day's responsibilities.

By **05:20**, she is driving through the nearly empty streets toward the regional children's hospital, the sky still dark as the hospital tower comes into view. After changing into scrubs and securing her badge, **Lauren Mitchell, RN, BSN, RNC-NIC** enters the NICU, where the environment feels markedly different from most hospital units—lights dimmed, voices quiet, and alarms carefully managed to reduce stimulation for fragile patients. The overnight nurse begins bedside report, detailing feeding schedules, ventilator settings, weight changes, medication timing, and subtle behavioral cues observed overnight.

Lauren receives two premature infants requiring continuous monitoring. The morning begins with careful assessments: checking incubator temperature settings, reviewing oxygen saturation trends, verifying feeding orders, and measuring tiny medication dosages that require absolute precision. NICU nursing demands meticulous attention to detail, as even small adjustments can significantly affect infant stability.

Parents begin arriving shortly after morning rounds. For many, the NICU experience is emotionally overwhelming—excitement about their newborn mixed with anxiety about medical uncertainty. Lauren greets them warmly, explains the overnight progress, and demonstrates how they can participate in care activities such as gentle touch or assisted feeding when appropriate. Teaching and emotional reassurance form a central part of neonatal nursing, helping families build confidence as their infants grow stronger.

Late morning involves feeding support, laboratory sample coordination, and collaboration with neonatologists, respiratory therapists, and lactation consultants. One infant requires respiratory adjustment following oxygen saturation fluctuations, and Lauren works closely with the respiratory therapist to fine-tune settings while monitoring the infant's response. Each adjustment is small but significant, requiring continuous observation afterward.

Throughout the afternoon, she documents feeding tolerance, weight measurements, medication administration, and developmental observations that guide care planning. The

NICU operates with a rhythm of careful monitoring rather than rapid activity, yet the level of vigilance remains constant. When an alarm sounds, the response is immediate but controlled, ensuring minimal disruption to surrounding infants.

As evening handoff approaches, Lauren prepares a detailed report for the incoming nurse—feeding volumes, medication schedules, parental education provided, and any clinical trends requiring attention overnight. Continuity of care is critical; infants often remain in the NICU for extended periods, and consistent communication supports steady progress.

Driving home after the shift, the emotional intensity of the unit lingers gently—thoughts of infants gaining weight, parents learning to hold their babies for the first time, and the gradual progress that defines neonatal recovery. At home, Willow greets her at the door, and the quiet evening routine begins—dinner, conversation, and a few moments of rest before another early morning when the NICU will again require patience, precision, and compassionate care.

SCRUB*fit*™ Hope Fulle, RN, BSN — Reflection

"Lauren's day is exactly why NICU nursing feels so distinct from the rest of the hospital — the pace is quiet, but the responsibility is immense, and the work is built on micro-decisions that carry macro consequences. Everything here is precision: incubator settings, oxygen saturation trends, feeding volumes, weight changes, tiny medication dosages that leave no room for casual math or 'close enough.' If a nurse feels calmer when the environment is controlled and the vigilance is sustained, this setting can feel deeply aligned, because you're not chasing chaos; you're protecting fragility. What also stands out is the emotional steadiness required

with families. Parents arrive carrying a storm of feelings, and the NICU nurse becomes both translator and anchor — explaining the clinical picture in a way that doesn't inflate fear, while also never minimizing reality. Lauren's shift shows the NICU rhythm: careful assessments, measured adjustments, deliberate responses to alarms, and documentation that captures not only medical data but developmental nuance and parental progress. Nurses who need fast turnover, constant novelty, or high-volume interaction may feel constrained here, but nurses who are wired for patience, continuity, and meticulous care often find this work profoundly sustaining. In the NICU, improvement is incremental and hard-earned — and that slow, steady progress is exactly what makes the job feel meaningful."

Chapter 20

Day In The Life — Oncology Unit

David Nguyen, RN, BSN, OCN wakes at **05:25**, the soft morning light beginning to fill the apartment. His coffee maker clicks on automatically, a small convenience he set the night before, and the gentle sound wakes his elderly beagle, Rosie, who slowly pads into the kitchen expecting breakfast. David pours coffee, prepares oatmeal, and checks the oncology unit staffing message on his phone—several chemotherapy infusions scheduled, one new admission, and two patients preparing for discharge later in the afternoon.

After feeding Rosie and taking her briefly outside, he gathers his lunch bag and heads out for the thirty-minute commute to the hospital's cancer center. The drive offers a few quiet minutes to mentally prepare for the emotional tone of oncology nursing, where long-term patient relationships often form and conversations extend beyond immediate clinical care.

Inside the oncology unit, **David Nguyen, RN, BSN, OCN** receives report on four patients. Two are receiving scheduled chemotherapy treatments, one is recovering from a recent surgical procedure related to cancer treatment, and another is admitted for symptom management. Oncology nursing combines technical medication administration with significant patient education, requiring careful attention to treatment protocols and supportive care measures.

Morning assessments begin with reviewing lab results that determine whether chemotherapy can proceed safely. David checks blood counts, verifies physician orders, and confirms medication preparation with the pharmacy before initiating infusions. Chemotherapy administration involves strict safety protocols, and each step—from patient identification to infusion monitoring—requires double verification to ensure accuracy.

Throughout the morning, he monitors patients closely for side effects, adjusts supportive medications as ordered, and answers patient and family questions about treatment expectations. Many oncology patients return for repeated treatments over months or years, creating ongoing relationships between nurses and families. Conversations often include not only clinical updates but also encouragement, reassurance, and discussion about coping strategies during treatment.

Afternoon hours involve discharge planning for a patient completing a treatment cycle. David reviews medication schedules, hydration recommendations, and signs that require medical attention once at home. Education is detailed, ensuring patients feel confident managing side effects and understanding follow-up appointment timelines. Nearby, a new patient admission requires orientation to the unit, explanation of treatment schedules, and emotional reassurance during an understandably stressful time.

Documentation remains continuous—infusion start and stop times, patient tolerance, medication administration, and education notes all entered carefully into the electronic record. Oncology nursing emphasizes continuity, as accurate records guide future treatment cycles and physician decision-making.

As evening approaches, David prepares handoff report for the incoming nurse, reviewing lab trends, infusion schedules, symptom management plans, and family concerns that may require attention overnight. Clear communication ensures ongoing treatments continue safely without interruption.

Driving home at sunset, he reflects on the steady pace of oncology nursing—less dramatic than emergency care yet deeply impactful over time. At home, Rosie greets him enthusiastically, tail wagging despite her slower pace, and the evening transitions into dinner, a short neighborhood walk, and quiet rest before the next shift caring for patients navigating long and often challenging treatment journeys.

Chapter 21

Day In The Life — Physician Office

Carla Simmons, RN, BSN wakes at **06:10**, the later start compared to her previous hospital roles still feeling like a small luxury. Morning sunlight filters through the kitchen window as she pours coffee and feeds her two cats, Jasper and Lila, who circle the food bowls with predictable enthusiasm. Breakfast is quick—toast, fruit, and coffee—before she reviews the day's clinic schedule on her phone: annual physicals, chronic disease follow-ups, several immunizations, and a handful of same-day urgent appointments added overnight.

Her fifteen-minute drive to the primary care clinic passes quickly, morning traffic moving steadily through the suburban streets. After arriving and logging into the clinic system, **Carla Simmons, RN, BSN** begins preparing exam rooms—restocking supplies, checking vaccine inventory, and reviewing patient charts for any flagged notes or pending lab results that physicians may need during visits.

The first patients begin arriving shortly after the clinic opens. Carla escorts them from the waiting room, verifies medications, updates health histories, and records vital signs before the physician enters. Physician-office nursing blends clinical assessment with patient education and care coordination, often serving as the first point of contact for patient concerns. One patient asks questions about newly prescribed blood pressure medication, and Carla reviews dosing instructions and potential side effects before documenting the conversation in the chart.

Mid-morning brings a steady rhythm of immunizations, wound checks, and follow-up visits for chronic conditions such as diabetes and asthma. Carla coordinates lab orders, schedules referrals, and communicates with pharmacies regarding prescription clarifications. Unlike hospital settings where care focuses on acute illness, clinic nursing emphasizes prevention, long-term disease management, and helping patients navigate the broader healthcare system.

Late morning includes a same-day urgent appointment for a patient experiencing respiratory symptoms. Carla performs the intake assessment, collects preliminary testing samples, and prepares the exam room for the provider, ensuring the visit proceeds efficiently. Communication remains constant—between physicians, medical assistants, laboratory staff, and front-desk teams—keeping patient flow smooth throughout the day.

After a short lunch break, the afternoon schedule continues with routine visits and discharge teaching. Carla spends time explaining lifestyle modifications to a patient newly diagnosed with diabetes, reviewing nutrition resources, home monitoring instructions, and follow-up appointment timelines. Education plays a central role in physician-office nursing, where the goal is often to prevent conditions from worsening before hospitalization becomes necessary.

As the final appointments conclude, Carla completes charting, confirms lab orders have been transmitted, and prepares exam rooms for the next day's schedule. Compared to hospital shifts, the clinic closes with a predictable end time, allowing staff to leave once patient care and documentation are complete.

Driving home in the late afternoon, she reflects on the quieter but equally meaningful rhythm of outpatient nursing—helping patients manage health over months and years rather than only during acute illness. At home, Jasper and Lila greet her at the door, the evening settling into a relaxed routine of dinner, reading, and a walk around the neighborhood before another clinic day begins tomorrow.

SCRUB*fit*™ Suzette Soleil, RN — Reflection

"Carla's day isn't med-surg in the literal sense, but the rhythm she's living in the clinic is very familiar to me: steady throughput, constant coordination, and a whole lot of quiet prioritizing that never really stops. Instead of five inpatient rooms, she's managing a rolling panel of needs — vitals, med reconciliation, immunizations, chart flags, labs, referrals, pharmacy clarifications, and those same-day urgent add-ons that drop into the schedule like surprise admissions. What I notice most is how outpatient nursing trades acute intensity for long-game impact. You're not titrating drips or juggling discharges, but you are preventing the hospitalization that happens later if education doesn't land today. That requires a

different kind of stamina: patience, repetition, and the ability to teach clearly even when you're on visit number fourteen and the phone is ringing again.

This setting is deeply aligned for nurses who like operational flow, clean systems, and the satisfaction of closing loops — making sure the lab order actually went through, the referral actually got scheduled, the patient actually understands what 'take with food' means, and the vaccine inventory is right before tomorrow hits. If a nurse needs the adrenaline of inpatient unpredictability or feels most motivated by crisis response, clinic work can feel too quiet or too routine. But if you're wired for consistency, prevention, and practical problem-solving across a whole day of small decisions, outpatient nursing can be surprisingly sustaining — because the work ends with a real sense of completion, and the outcomes show up over months and years. Carla's shift is a reminder that nursing isn't only about what you do in the hospital; it's about whether the pace and purpose of the day match how you're built."

Chapter 22

Day In The Life — Home Health Nurse

Here is a **Home Health Nurse — Day-in-the-Life Dispatch** you can use.

Home Health Nurse — Day-in-the-Life Dispatch

06:15 — The morning begins quietly. Maria Lopez, RN, BSN wakes to the soft buzz of her alarm and the low snoring of her miniature schnauzer, Rico, curled at the foot of the bed. Unlike hospital nursing, where the shift begins the moment you badge in, home health nursing starts with planning. Coffee brews while Maria opens her tablet at the kitchen table, reviewing the day's route: five patient visits across three neighborhoods, each requiring a different type of care — wound management, medication reconciliation, chronic disease monitoring, and a new-admission assessment scheduled for late afternoon.

Breakfast is quick — oatmeal, fruit, and coffee — while she checks traffic patterns and confirms appointment windows through the agency's scheduling system. Home health nursing blends clinical care with logistical coordination, and route efficiency can make the difference between a smooth day and a stressful one. By **07:10**, she loads her supply bag into the car: gloves, wound kits, portable vital-sign monitor, documentation tablet, and backup PPE. Rico watches from the front window as she pulls away, the quiet neighborhood just beginning to wake.

08:00 – The first visit is a post-surgical patient recovering from a knee replacement. Inside the patient's home, the pace immediately feels different from the hospital. There are no overhead pages, no constant alarms – just the everyday rhythm of someone's living space. Maria begins with a friendly greeting, washes her hands at the kitchen sink, and sets up a small clean field for wound care supplies. She checks vital signs, assesses mobility progress, and carefully changes the dressing while reviewing physical therapy exercises the patient is expected to complete later that day. Education is constant in home health nursing; each visit is both treatment and coaching session, helping patients safely manage recovery between professional visits.

09:15 – The next stop is a diabetic patient requiring blood-glucose monitoring review and medication adjustment follow-up. Maria confirms medication adherence, reviews recent readings, and discusses diet modifications recommended by the primary care provider. Unlike inpatient settings where meals are controlled, home environments reveal the real-life barriers patients face – limited grocery access, mobility issues, or confusion about medication timing. Problem-solving becomes part of clinical care, and Maria spends a few extra minutes helping the patient set reminder alarms on their phone to support medication consistency.

10:30 – Driving between visits provides brief moments of reset. The car becomes a mobile office where she dictates quick documentation notes through voice entry before heading to the next home. The third visit involves an elderly patient recently discharged after pneumonia treatment. Maria performs respiratory assessment, reviews inhaler technique, and ensures follow-up appointments are scheduled. A family member joins the conversation, asking questions about warning signs that should prompt a call to the physician. These discussions often prevent hospital readmissions, making home health nurses key players in continuity-of-care systems.

12:00 – Lunch happens in the car between neighborhoods – a packed sandwich, fruit, and water – while she confirms the afternoon schedule. Flexibility is essential; patients occasionally need rescheduling due to physician appointments, transportation delays, or unexpected health changes. Today's fourth visit, a wound-care follow-up, requires extra preparation, so Maria reviews prior photos and measurements to compare healing progress before arrival.

13:00 – At the fourth home, she performs a detailed wound assessment, measures healing margins, updates photographs for the clinical record, and communicates progress to the supervising provider through the agency's system. Home health nursing often requires autonomous clinical judgment within defined protocols, and accurate documentation ensures that physicians can adjust care plans without requiring patients to travel back to clinics unnecessarily.

14:45 — The final visit of the day is a new patient admission. These appointments are longer and involve comprehensive assessment — medication reconciliation, home safety evaluation, baseline vitals, fall-risk screening, and patient education about how home health services will function. Maria checks for environmental risks such as loose rugs, poor lighting, or inaccessible medication storage, offering small but practical suggestions that can significantly reduce injury risk. She reviews emergency contact procedures and explains how to reach the agency after hours if symptoms change.

16:30 — With visits completed, Maria spends time parked in a quiet lot finishing documentation. Home health nursing requires real-time charting to ensure accuracy, especially when coordinating with physicians, therapists, and case managers who rely on those notes to plan next steps. Once records are finalized, she confirms tomorrow's tentative route and checks supply levels to determine what needs restocking at the office.

17:15 — The drive home signals the mental transition out of clinical mode. Unlike hospital shifts that end with unit handoff, home health nurses carry a sense of completion tied to each individual visit — each home entered, each patient stabilized, each teaching moment delivered. Traffic is heavier now, but the steady rhythm of the commute provides a welcome pause.

18:00 — Back home, Rico greets her enthusiastically at the door, leash already in mouth for the evening walk. After a short stroll around the neighborhood, Maria prepares dinner and briefly reflects on the day's progress: a surgical wound healing well, a patient gaining confidence with insulin management, a new admission safely oriented to care services. Home health nursing may lack the visible urgency of hospital units, but its impact is measured in something equally powerful — helping patients remain safely in their homes while continuing recovery.

By the time evening settles in, supplies are repacked for the next day, the schedule is reviewed once more, and the quiet preparation that defines home health nursing begins again — a profession built not on a single central workplace, but on dozens of front doors where clinical skill, independence, and patient education come together to support healing in everyday life.

SCRUB*fit*™ Suzette Soleil, RN — Reflection

Maria's day reminds me that nursing isn't defined by the building you work in — it's defined by the coordination, prioritization, and patient-centered problem-solving that follow you wherever care happens. In home health, the patient list isn't down a hallway; it's spread across neighborhoods, and every visit requires you to reset, reassess, and adapt to a completely different environment. What stands out most is the autonomy. There's no immediate team at the bedside, which means your clinical judgment, preparation, and teaching skills carry even more weight. Nurses who thrive on independence, relationship-based care, and the satisfaction of helping patients manage real-life recovery challenges often feel deeply aligned in home health. At the same time, nurses who prefer the constant collaboration and immediate backup of a hospital unit may feel isolated by the solo nature of the work. The rhythm is different — less visible urgency, more long-term stabilization — but the impact is enormous. Every clear teaching moment, every medication clarification, and every safety adjustment inside a patient's home quietly prevents complications later, and that kind of steady, preventative care is a powerful form of nursing leadership in action.

Chapter 23

Alternative Practice Environments™ — Careers for the Adventurous

While most people associate Registered Nursing with hospitals, clinics, and traditional care settings, the nursing credential is far more geographically and operationally flexible than many early-career professionals initially realize. Around the world, healthcare organizations, government agencies, private expedition groups, humanitarian teams, maritime medical services, and remote-industry employers rely on nurses who are willing to work in environments that combine clinical care with travel, unpredictability, and operational independence. These roles are not designed for everyone; they often require flexibility, resilience, additional certifications, and comfort operating with limited immediate backup. For nurses drawn to exploration, cultural immersion, or unconventional work environments, however, these practice settings can create uniquely fulfilling career pathways that extend far beyond traditional clinical roles.

Adventure-oriented nursing roles share several common characteristics. Work environments are frequently mobile or remote, resources may be limited compared with hospital settings, and clinical decision-making often requires heightened independence and adaptability. Nurses in these roles must rely heavily on assessment skills, stabilization techniques, and communication with remote medical directors or transport teams when escalation is necessary. Because patient access to higher-level care may involve transportation delays, early recognition of deterioration and decisive intervention become especially critical. Many nurses who transition into these roles describe them as combining the clinical focus of nursing practice with the situational awareness and operational planning found in emergency response fields. The result is a professional environment that blends healthcare expertise with logistical problem-solving and situational adaptability.

Expedition and Wilderness Nursing

Expedition and wilderness medicine roles place nurses in some of the most remote environments on earth, including mountain expeditions, polar research stations, remote eco-tourism programs, scientific field teams, and wilderness education organizations. In these environments, nurses frequently serve as the primary on-site healthcare professional responsible for initial assessment, stabilization, and coordination of evacuation when necessary. Clinical encounters may range from altitude illness and environmental exposure injuries to orthopedic trauma, dehydration, or acute medical conditions that occur far from hospital infrastructure. Because evacuation logistics can involve hours or even days depending on terrain and weather conditions, strong triage judgment and stabilization capability are essential competencies.

Nurses entering wilderness roles often pursue additional training such as wilderness medicine certification, remote trauma courses, or advanced emergency care programs that emphasize field improvisation, environmental physiology, and prolonged patient care scenarios. The work schedule is typically structured around expedition cycles rather than traditional shift rotations, meaning assignments may involve extended deployments followed by periods of time off. Professionals drawn to outdoor environments, travel, and autonomous clinical decision-making frequently find these roles professionally rewarding, particularly when they value experiential diversity over predictable scheduling structures. While compensation varies depending on organization type, the experiential value and professional uniqueness of the work attract nurses seeking careers that combine healthcare with exploration.

Event and Mass-Gathering Medical Support

Large-scale public events—including concerts, festivals, endurance races, professional sporting events, and international conventions—require dedicated medical support teams capable of managing high patient volumes within compressed timeframes. Registered Nurses play essential roles within these event-medicine teams, providing triage, first-line treatment, hydration management, minor trauma care, and coordination with emergency medical transport units when hospital transfer becomes necessary. Event medicine environments are dynamic, fast-paced, and heavily teamwork-oriented, often resembling emergency department workflow patterns compressed into temporary care environments. Patient presentations commonly include dehydration, heat-related illness, intoxication-related complications, minor injuries, and occasionally higher-acuity emergencies requiring rapid stabilization.

Many nurses participate in event medical coverage as supplemental work assignments or seasonal engagements, while others develop long-term involvement with event-medicine organizations that operate nationally or internationally. These roles allow nurses to combine clinical practice with travel opportunities, exposure to diverse operational settings, and participation in large-scale public safety planning. Event medicine also strengthens triage efficiency, rapid assessment skills, and interdisciplinary coordination abilities, competencies that translate effectively back into hospital environments. For nurses seeking flexible, episodic clinical work that introduces variety into their professional routines, event medical support can become a compelling adjunct or alternative practice pathway.

Cruise Ship and Maritime Nursing

Cruise ship medicine represents another distinctive practice environment where nurses provide healthcare services to both passengers and crew members while operating in international maritime settings. Shipboard medical centers function as compact clinical units capable of handling routine illnesses, urgent care needs, minor procedures, and stabilization of patients requiring evacuation to shore-based hospitals when necessary. Nurses in these roles manage patient assessments, medication administration, clinical documentation, emergency response participation, and coordination with ship command structures during health-related incidents. Because ships operate outside immediate hospital access for extended periods, clinical teams must maintain strong emergency-preparedness protocols and telemedicine communication with consulting physicians when required.

Maritime nursing roles often appeal to professionals interested in international travel combined with structured employment assignments that may last several months at a time. While schedules can be demanding during active voyages, many positions include extended off-contract periods between assignments, allowing professionals to balance intensive work intervals with personal travel or rest periods. Nurses considering maritime roles typically benefit from prior acute-care experience, emergency response familiarity, and strong independent clinical decision-making ability. The global exposure and operational uniqueness of shipboard healthcare delivery create professional experiences rarely encountered in traditional clinical environments.

Humanitarian and Global Health Missions

Humanitarian medical missions and international relief deployments represent another pathway for nurses interested in combining clinical practice with global service. Non-governmental organizations, disaster-response agencies, and international health initiatives frequently deploy nurses to regions affected by natural disasters, conflict-related displacement, infectious disease outbreaks, or infrastructure disruptions. Clinical responsibilities may include emergency care, vaccination campaigns, maternal-child health support, community health education, and collaboration with international medical teams operating under resource-limited conditions. These roles demand adaptability, cross-cultural communication skills, and the ability to deliver effective care despite supply limitations or rapidly changing operational environments.

Participation in humanitarian work can occur through short-term volunteer assignments, rotational global-health employment programs, or long-term organizational roles focused on international public-health initiatives. Many nurses find these experiences deeply meaningful because they allow direct engagement with global health challenges while expanding professional perspective beyond domestic healthcare systems. Exposure to diverse care delivery models often strengthens clinical creativity, cultural awareness, and leadership capacity, skills that continue to influence professional practice long after returning to traditional clinical environments. While these roles require preparation, training, and thoughtful organizational selection, they offer opportunities to apply nursing expertise in ways that directly impact underserved populations worldwide.

Mobile Health, Travel Contracts, and Remote Industry Roles

Adventure-aligned practice environments also include domestic travel nursing assignments, remote industrial healthcare roles such as offshore energy platforms or remote construction sites, and mobile health programs serving rural or underserved communities. Travel nursing positions allow Registered Nurses to accept time-limited contracts across different regions, experiencing varied clinical environments while often receiving housing assistance or travel stipends. Remote industrial health positions frequently involve providing occupational health support, emergency stabilization capability, and health-promotion services for workforce populations operating far from urban medical centers. Mobile health units similarly extend care access into communities lacking consistent clinic infrastructure, allowing nurses to deliver screenings, preventive care services, and chronic-disease management support directly within community settings.

These roles appeal to professionals seeking geographic mobility, variety in clinical exposure, or opportunities to combine healthcare practice with broader operational environments. The adaptability developed through working across diverse care settings often enhances long-term professional versatility, enabling nurses to transition between specialties more easily over the course of their careers. For individuals who value flexibility, experiential diversity, and professional mobility, these practice environments represent powerful alternatives to fixed-location clinical roles. Over time, many nurses integrate periods of traditional hospital practice with intervals of travel or remote assignments, creating career trajectories that balance stability with exploration.

Who Thrives in Adventure-Oriented Nursing Roles

Not every nurse is drawn to unconventional environments, and these roles are not inherently "better" than traditional clinical pathways; they simply align more closely with certain professional preferences and personality profiles. Nurses who thrive in these environments typically demonstrate comfort with independence, adaptability to changing conditions, strong assessment skills, and enthusiasm for travel or nontraditional work structures. They often value experiential variety over highly predictable scheduling and enjoy problem-solving in environments where resources may be limited or logistical challenges require creative solutions. Professionals who prefer tightly structured workflows, immediate access to specialty consultation, or highly predictable scheduling patterns may find traditional hospital roles more aligned with their preferences.

Understanding these differences is important because career satisfaction often depends less on compensation alone and more on alignment between professional environment and personal temperament. Adventure-oriented practice pathways expand the visible horizon of what nursing careers can look like, reminding professionals that licensure does not restrict them to a single environment for the entirety of their careers. Many nurses spend portions of their professional journey exploring alternative practice settings before returning to long-term specialty roles, while others build entire careers around mobile or international healthcare delivery. The flexibility of the nursing profession allows both approaches to coexist, enabling individuals to design career paths that reflect both professional goals and lifestyle preferences over time.

Chapter 24

Alternative Practice Environments™ — Pathways, Preparation, and Entry Strategies

Exploring nontraditional nursing environments requires more than curiosity; it requires strategic preparation, credential planning, and a realistic understanding of how these roles are actually obtained. Unlike hospital-based hiring, which often follows standardized residency or recruitment pipelines, many alternative practice positions are secured through professional networking, specialty training organizations, contract staffing agencies, or direct outreach to expedition, maritime, humanitarian, and event-medicine employers. Nurses interested in these paths benefit from early exposure to emergency-care environments, independent decision-making experiences, and certifications that demonstrate readiness for field-based practice settings. Employers in these environments often prioritize demonstrated adaptability and operational readiness over purely academic credentials.

Building the Right Experience First

Most adventure-oriented practice roles expect candidates to have a foundation in acute-care environments such as emergency departments, critical care units, trauma services, or high-acuity medical-surgical settings. These clinical backgrounds build rapid-assessment capability, stabilization experience, and comfort managing unpredictable patient presentations—skills that become essential when working in remote or resource-limited environments. Nurses early in their careers can intentionally select first positions that strengthen these competencies if long-term interest in travel or expedition practice exists. Even two to three years of targeted acute-care experience can significantly expand eligibility for these specialized pathways. Strategic early-career planning therefore plays a major role in opening later nontraditional opportunities.

Certifications That Open Doors

Additional certifications often strengthen candidacy for alternative practice environments. Training programs in wilderness medicine, emergency trauma care, occupational health, advanced cardiac life support, pediatric advanced life support, or remote clinical response demonstrate preparedness for independent clinical operation. While not every position requires specialized certifications, many employers view them as indicators of readiness for environments where immediate specialist backup may not be available. Continuing education investments also signal professional initiative, a trait often valued in mobile or expedition-based roles where team members must operate with significant autonomy. Over time, nurses who build layered certification portfolios frequently gain access to a broader range of nontraditional assignments.

Networking and Opportunity Discovery

Many adventure-oriented nursing opportunities are not widely advertised through traditional hospital job boards. Instead, they circulate through professional associations, specialty staffing agencies, global health organizations, maritime employment networks, and word-of-mouth referrals within niche professional communities. Building relationships with colleagues who have participated in travel contracts, humanitarian deployments, or expedition medicine programs often becomes one of the most effective ways to learn about available roles. Professional conferences, specialty training programs, and online nursing communities can also provide exposure to organizations seeking clinicians for short-term or project-based assignments. Networking in these spaces is less about self-promotion and more about learning how these career ecosystems function operationally.

Financial and Lifestyle Planning

Adventure-oriented roles often involve compensation structures that differ from traditional hospital employment models. Some assignments offer premium short-term pay structures, while others prioritize experiential opportunities over financial incentives, particularly in humanitarian or volunteer-based deployments. Nurses considering these pathways benefit from evaluating both the financial and lifestyle implications of assignments, including travel schedules, housing arrangements, contract duration, and healthcare coverage provisions. Planning financially for variable assignment cycles ensures that mobility-focused careers remain sustainable over the long term. Professionals who approach these roles strategically often combine traditional employment periods with travel assignments to balance income stability and experiential goals.

Long-Term Career Integration

Participation in alternative practice environments does not require permanent departure from traditional clinical pathways. Many nurses rotate between hospital practice and travel-based assignments across different stages of their careers, allowing them to maintain specialty proficiency while periodically engaging in exploratory roles. Experiences gained through remote medicine, expedition care, or international health programs frequently strengthen clinical confidence, cultural competence, and leadership capabilities that later enhance hospital-based practice as well. Over time, this blend of structured clinical experience and exploratory assignments can produce highly adaptable professionals capable of functioning effectively across diverse care environments. The flexibility of nursing licensure allows careers to evolve dynamically rather than follow a single predetermined path.

Chapter 25

No One Told Me This About Nursing School

Many people begin nursing school believing the greatest challenge will be academic difficulty — mastering pharmacology, anatomy, physiology, and clinical theory at a level far beyond previous coursework. While the academic workload is significant, what surprises many students most is not the complexity of the material, but the pace and structure of the program itself. Nursing education compresses large volumes of information into accelerated timelines while simultaneously requiring clinical rotations that often begin early in the program. Students quickly discover that success depends not only on intelligence, but on time management, endurance, organization, and the ability to perform under sustained pressure. Programs are designed intentionally this way, because the realities of healthcare require clinicians who can function effectively even when workloads are heavy and environments are unpredictable. Understanding this structure early helps students prepare mentally before the first semester even begins.

Another unexpected reality involves clinical scheduling. Clinical rotations frequently begin at very early hours, sometimes requiring students to arrive at hospitals before sunrise to receive assignments and prepare for patient care activities. These schedules often shift each semester depending on rotation type, instructor availability, and clinical-site partnerships, making consistent weekly routines difficult to maintain. Many students enter programs expecting predictable academic timetables similar to traditional college courses, only to discover that nursing education operates more like a professional training environment than a conventional academic schedule. Work responsibilities, childcare arrangements, commuting logistics, and financial planning must often be adjusted repeatedly throughout the program. Those who anticipate these schedule fluctuations in advance tend to manage the transition more smoothly than those caught off guard by the variability.

Financial planning is another area where many students wish they had received clearer guidance before enrollment. Tuition is only one portion of the total cost of nursing education. Students frequently incur additional expenses for uniforms, equipment, licensing exams, background checks, transportation to clinical sites, certification courses such as basic life support, and sometimes unpaid clinical hours that reduce the ability to maintain full-time employment. While nursing offers strong long-term earning potential, the short-term financial strain during training can be significant if not planned carefully. Exploring scholarship programs, employer sponsorship opportunities, or part-time healthcare employment prior to enrollment can reduce long-term financial pressure. Financial awareness early in the process often makes the educational journey far more manageable.

Perhaps the most important lesson that many students discover only after beginning the program is that nursing school is not only an academic experience; it is an emotional training process. Clinical rotations introduce students to illness, trauma, recovery, and occasionally loss for the first time in close proximity. Even when instructors provide strong support, the emotional weight of witnessing real patient experiences can be heavier than many students initially expect. Learning to maintain professionalism while also developing emotional resilience becomes an essential skill that is not always discussed openly during admissions counseling. Students who build peer support networks, maintain personal wellness routines, and seek mentorship during challenging rotations often adapt more successfully than those who attempt to manage the experience entirely alone.

Finally, many students are surprised to learn that perfection is not the expectation in nursing education — growth is. Early mistakes, nervous clinical performances, and moments of uncertainty are common parts of the training process, and instructors expect students to improve progressively rather than perform flawlessly from the beginning. The programs are structured to build competence step by step, allowing students to develop confidence through repeated exposure and guided practice. Understanding this perspective can significantly reduce the anxiety many students feel during their first clinical experiences. Nursing education is not designed to identify perfect candidates; it is designed to develop capable professionals over time.

• • •

What I Wish I Had Known About Nursing

One of the most common reflections nurses share after entering the profession is that the first job matters more than the first specialty. Many new graduates focus heavily on securing positions in highly competitive units immediately after graduation, believing that long-term career success depends on starting in a specific environment. In reality, the most important early-career factor is often the quality of orientation, mentorship, and leadership support provided by the hiring organization. Strong onboarding programs build clinical confidence and long-term retention, while weak orientation environments can create unnecessary stress even for highly capable new graduates. Evaluating the strength of residency programs, mentorship availability, and turnover rates within units can provide more valuable insight than focusing solely on prestige or specialty titles.

Another insight many nurses discover only after entering the workforce is that time management becomes a clinical skill, not just a personal productivity technique. Nursing shifts require simultaneous coordination of medication schedules, patient assessments, interdisciplinary communication, documentation, and unexpected patient needs that arise without warning. Learning to prioritize dynamically—adjusting plans as conditions change—becomes essential for maintaining both patient safety and personal workflow efficiency. While nursing school introduces these concepts, real-world practice sharpens them significantly, and new nurses often report that mastering prioritization was one of the most transformative skills they developed during their first year. Early awareness of this reality helps graduates approach orientation periods with more realistic expectations.

Compensation and scheduling realities also surprise many new nurses. While the profession offers strong income stability, total earnings often vary based on shift differentials, overtime availability, specialty environments, and geographic location. Some nurses discover that night shifts or weekend rotations significantly influence early-career income, while others find that schedule flexibility becomes more valuable than incremental pay differences as personal responsibilities evolve. Understanding how compensation structures actually function helps nurses make more informed decisions about early career opportunities rather than focusing only on base salary numbers. Financial planning within nursing benefits from viewing career progression as a multi-year trajectory rather than a single job decision.

Another lesson frequently shared involves the importance of career flexibility. Nursing education prepares graduates for entry-level clinical roles, but the profession contains far more pathways than many students initially realize. Over time, nurses transition into specialties such as critical care, procedural environments, community health, leadership, education, informatics, and advanced practice roles depending on interests and life priorities. Recognizing that career evolution is expected—not exceptional—helps reduce the pressure many new nurses feel to make "perfect" early-career decisions. The first role is rarely permanent; it is the foundation upon which future opportunities are built.

Perhaps the most meaningful reflection nurses share is that confidence develops gradually, not instantly at graduation. The first months of professional practice often feel overwhelming, even for high-performing students, because responsibility increases dramatically once independent licensure begins. With consistent experience, supportive mentorship, and repeated clinical exposure, the uncertainty gradually gives way to steady competence. Nurses who understand this developmental curve early tend to remain more patient with themselves during the transition from student to practicing professional. Over time, the tasks that once required intense concentration become routine, allowing greater focus on advanced clinical judgment and patient advocacy. The profession rewards persistence, and those who remain engaged through the early learning curve often discover a level of professional confidence they once doubted they could achieve.

Chapter 26
What I Wish I Had Known About Nursing

One of the most common reflections nurses share after entering the profession is that the **first job matters more than the first specialty**. Many new graduates focus heavily on securing positions in highly competitive units immediately after graduation, believing that long-term career success depends on starting in a specific environment. In reality, the most important early-career factor is often the quality of orientation, mentorship, and leadership support provided by the hiring organization. Strong onboarding programs build clinical confidence and long-term retention, while weak orientation environments can create unnecessary stress even for highly capable new graduates. Evaluating the strength of residency programs, mentorship availability, and turnover rates within units can provide more valuable insight than focusing solely on prestige or specialty titles.

Another insight many nurses discover only after entering the workforce is that **time management becomes a clinical skill**, not just a personal productivity technique. Nursing shifts require simultaneous coordination of medication schedules, patient assessments, interdisciplinary communication, documentation, and unexpected patient needs that arise without warning. Learning to prioritize dynamically—adjusting plans as conditions change—becomes essential for maintaining both patient safety and personal workflow efficiency. While nursing school introduces these concepts, real-world practice sharpens them significantly, and new nurses often report that mastering prioritization was one of the most transformative skills they developed during their first year. Early awareness of this reality helps graduates approach orientation periods with more realistic expectations.

Compensation and scheduling realities also surprise many new nurses. While the profession offers strong income stability, total earnings often vary based on shift differentials, overtime availability, specialty environments, and geographic location. Some nurses discover that night shifts or weekend rotations significantly influence early-career income, while others find that schedule flexibility becomes more valuable than incremental pay differences as personal responsibilities evolve. Understanding how compensation structures actually function helps nurses make more informed decisions about early career opportunities rather than focusing only on base salary numbers. Financial planning within nursing benefits from viewing career progression as a multi-year trajectory rather than a single job decision.

Another lesson frequently shared involves the importance of **career flexibility**. Nursing education prepares graduates for entry-level clinical roles, but the profession contains far more pathways than many students initially realize. Over time, nurses transition into specialties such as critical care, procedural environments, community health, leadership, education, informatics, and advanced practice roles depending on interests and life priorities. Recognizing that career evolution is expected—not exceptional—helps reduce the pressure many new nurses feel to make "perfect" early-career decisions. The first role is rarely permanent; it is the foundation upon which future opportunities are built.

Perhaps the most meaningful reflection nurses share is that **confidence develops gradually**, not instantly at graduation. The first months of professional practice often feel overwhelming, even for high-performing students, because responsibility increases dramatically once independent licensure begins. With consistent experience, supportive mentorship, and repeated clinical exposure, the uncertainty gradually gives way to steady competence. Nurses who understand this developmental curve early tend to remain more patient with themselves during the transition from student to practicing professional. Over time, the tasks that once required intense concentration become routine, allowing greater focus on advanced clinical judgment and patient advocacy. The profession rewards persistence, and those who remain engaged through the early learning curve often discover a level of professional confidence they once doubted they could achieve.

Chapter 27

CareerNav™

Hospitals do not hire nurses the way most applicants think they do.

From the outside, the process appears straightforward: job postings go live, candidates apply, interviews are scheduled, and offers follow. Inside healthcare systems, however, hiring is influenced by staffing ratios, budget cycles, seasonal census patterns, internal transfer pipelines, residency program commitments, and organizational approval layers that applicants rarely see. Understanding these forces does not make the process easier, but it does make it more predictable—and predictability is one of the most powerful advantages a job seeker can have.

Many nursing roles are effectively filled before the public posting ever gains attention. Internal candidates seeking unit transfers, staff members completing residency programs, float-pool nurses moving into permanent placements, and referral-based applicants often enter the hiring pipeline earlier than external applicants realize. Public listings frequently serve as compliance requirements or talent-pool collection points rather than true starting lines of the hiring process. This does not mean external candidates lack opportunity; it simply means they must approach the search more strategically.

Effective RN job searching operates across three parallel tracks. The first is **direct health-system career portals**, which reveal the most accurate picture of which specialties are expanding, which units repeatedly reopen postings, and which geographic locations demonstrate consistent demand. Repeated listings for the same specialty often signal structural turnover or rapid service growth—both indicators that hiring managers may be more open to candidates who demonstrate preparation and persistence.

The second track involves **residency and specialty-transition pipelines**. Many hospitals allocate a significant portion of their hiring capacity to structured new-graduate residency programs or internal cross-training initiatives. Nurses seeking entry into competitive specialties such as ICU, NICU, OR, or procedural areas often gain faster access through these structured pathways than through direct external applications. Understanding which systems offer formal transition programs can dramatically shorten the time required to move into desired specialties.

The third track is **relationship-based visibility**. Recruiters, nurse managers, clinical educators, and preceptors frequently maintain informal awareness lists of promising candidates encountered through clinical rotations, professional associations, volunteer work, or internal referrals. Candidates who maintain professional visibility—through clinical excellence during rotations, thoughtful follow-up communication, or participation in specialty organizations—often surface more quickly when openings occur, even before broad advertising begins.

Hiring timelines in nursing also fluctuate based on operational realities. Units experiencing sudden census increases may accelerate hiring decisions, while others may slow approvals temporarily due to budget reviews or staffing adjustments. Applicants sometimes interpret these fluctuations as personal rejection when they are actually system-level timing changes. Consistent follow-up, continued applications across multiple facilities, and maintaining multiple active opportunities helps stabilize momentum during these cycles.

Career navigation in nursing therefore becomes less about submitting a single perfect application and more about managing a **portfolio of opportunities**—tracking postings across systems, maintaining recruiter relationships, applying to multiple specialties aligned with long-term goals, and remaining attentive to residency or transition program deadlines. Over time, this layered approach significantly increases the likelihood of securing roles that match both career aspirations and personal lifestyle preferences.

Chapter 28

SCRUBScript™

Hiring managers reviewing Registered Nurse applications are rarely trying to determine whether candidates care about patients. Nearly every applicant entering the profession expresses dedication, compassion, and teamwork. What differentiates candidates is not intention—it is clarity, specificity, and evidence of readiness. A strong RN resume does not attempt to sound impressive; it demonstrates how the applicant is already functioning in ways that resemble the role being sought.

For new graduate nurses, the most important section of the resume is often clinical training. Instead of listing rotations as brief academic requirements, they should be presented as hands-on clinical experiences that demonstrate exposure to patient care responsibilities. Including unit type, approximate patient volume exposure, key procedures observed or assisted with, and electronic health record systems used helps hiring managers quickly understand the applicant's level of familiarity with clinical workflows. Even small details—such as participation in interdisciplinary rounds, patient education involvement, or assisting with medication administration under supervision—signal readiness to transition into professional practice.

Experienced Registered Nurses should shift emphasis from training exposure to measurable responsibilities and outcomes. Hiring managers look for indicators of assignment complexity, patient acuity levels, committee participation, preceptor roles, charge nurse responsibilities, and involvement in quality-improvement initiatives. These elements demonstrate operational contribution beyond routine patient care and signal professional growth within the clinical environment. Whenever possible, experience statements should reflect scope rather than general duties for example, referencing patient ratios, specialized equipment used, or interdisciplinary coordination responsibilities.

Resume formatting also influences how applications move through Applicant Tracking Systems (ATS). Simple layouts, consistent headings, and clear chronological structure allow systems to parse credentials accurately. Licensure and certifications should appear prominently near the top of the document, ensuring that reviewers immediately confirm eligibility. Many healthcare systems filter applicants based on license status, required certifications, or specialty keywords, making accurate placement of these elements essential.

Professional summaries should remain concise and factual rather than aspirational. Statements such as "Dedicated nurse seeking a challenging opportunity" rarely influence hiring decisions because they appear on thousands of applications. Instead, summaries should briefly describe licensure status, specialty exposure, and core competencies relevant to the target role—for example, experience in telemetry monitoring, perioperative preparation, or pediatric patient education. This approach communicates readiness rather than intention.

Another important component of RN resume strategy is customization. While maintaining a master resume is useful, tailoring select sections to reflect the language and competencies emphasized in each posting improves alignment with both ATS systems and hiring manager expectations. If a role emphasizes patient education, discharge planning, or procedural preparation, those elements should appear clearly within relevant experience descriptions rather than remaining buried in generalized statements.

Finally, resume effectiveness increases when it aligns with the broader hiring strategy. Applications submitted through internal referrals, residency pipelines, or recruiter introductions often receive faster review when the resume clearly reflects the competencies associated with the target unit. When hiring managers can quickly see how an applicant's preparation connects to their department's workflow, the application moves from "possible" to "interview-worthy" far more quickly.

A well-constructed RN resume therefore functions less as a biography and more as an operational snapshot—demonstrating licensure readiness, clinical exposure, assignment capability, and professional development in a format that allows reviewers to assess fit within seconds. In highly competitive hiring environments, that clarity often determines whether the application advances to the interview stage.

Chapter 29

Intelligent Interviews™

Nursing interviews are rarely designed to test whether you understand basic clinical tasks. Hiring managers assume that licensure, training, and clinical rotations have already established foundational competency. Instead, interviews are structured to evaluate how you think, how you respond under pressure, how you communicate with patients and teams, and how reliably you function when conditions become unpredictable. This is why many healthcare organizations rely heavily on **behavioral interviewing**—a format that asks candidates to describe how they handled real situations rather than how they *think* they would respond hypothetically.

Behavioral interviewing is based on a simple premise: past behavior is the best predictor of future performance. Rather than asking, "What would you do if a patient's condition changed suddenly?" interviewers ask, "Tell me about a time when you recognized a change in a patient's condition and what actions you took." The goal is to hear how candidates recognized the situation, prioritized tasks, communicated with the team, and followed through on patient care responsibilities.

A structured response approach helps candidates deliver clear answers. One widely used method is the **STAR framework**—Situation, Task, Action, Result. The Situation briefly explains the context. The Task clarifies the responsibility you held. The Action describes the specific steps you took. The Result explains what happened afterward and what you learned. Using this structure keeps responses focused and prevents candidates from drifting into unrelated details.

For example, a medication safety question might sound like:

"Tell me about a time when you caught a potential error or prevented a safety issue."

A strong response would briefly describe the clinical setting, identify the potential issue noticed, explain the verification steps taken, describe how the concern was communicated to the provider or team, and conclude with the outcome—whether the order was corrected, clarified, or adjusted. Interviewers are less interested in dramatic stories than in evidence of careful thinking, verification habits, and willingness to speak up for patient safety.

Another common behavioral topic involves teamwork.

"Describe a time when you had to collaborate with a difficult team member or manage a conflict on the unit."

In answering, interviewers listen for professionalism, communication style, and ability to maintain patient-centered focus rather than interpersonal frustration. Responses that show calm problem-solving, respectful escalation when necessary, and continued commitment to patient care demonstrate maturity and reliability.

Time management questions also appear frequently.

"Tell me about a time when you had multiple competing priorities and how you handled them."

Strong answers highlight prioritization decisions, use of delegation when appropriate, communication with the care team, and the final outcome of those decisions. Interviewers want to see that candidates can organize tasks logically without becoming overwhelmed when patient needs shift unexpectedly.

Clinical judgment questions may explore patient assessment awareness:

"Describe a situation where you noticed something subtle that others initially missed."

These responses allow candidates to demonstrate observational skills, escalation processes, and follow-up actions that protected patient safety. Even experiences from clinical rotations, internships, or early career assignments can provide meaningful examples when described clearly.

Preparation for behavioral interviews involves more than memorizing answers. Candidates benefit from identifying several real clinical scenarios in advance—patient safety moments, teamwork experiences, communication challenges, teaching interactions, and situations requiring rapid prioritization. Having these examples mentally organized allows flexibility during interviews because the same experience can often be adapted to answer multiple types of questions.

Interviewers also pay close attention to reflection. Candidates who briefly explain what they learned from an experience signal self-awareness and professional growth. Nursing leaders recognize that every clinician encounters challenging situations; what distinguishes strong professionals is their ability to evaluate those moments and apply lessons moving forward.

Finally, strong interview performance includes thoughtful candidate questions. Asking about orientation structure, mentorship opportunities, patient acuity expectations, or how the unit supports new nurses demonstrates genuine engagement with the role. Interviews function as two-way evaluations—the organization assesses the candidate, and the candidate evaluates whether the environment supports long-term success.

Behavioral interviewing therefore measures more than knowledge. It reveals how candidates think, communicate, prioritize, and respond to real-world clinical demands. When candidates prepare structured examples that demonstrate safe decision-making, teamwork, and reflective learning, interviews become opportunities to show readiness rather than moments of uncertainty.

Chapter 30

Saying Thank You™

The interview may feel like the final step in the hiring process, but the period immediately after the interview often influences hiring decisions more than many candidates realize. A brief, professional thank-you message reinforces interest in the role, demonstrates professionalism, and helps hiring teams remember candidates positively as they compare finalists. In highly competitive nursing markets, where several applicants may perform well during interviews, small professional gestures can become meaningful differentiators.

A thank-you message should be sent within twenty-four hours of the interview whenever possible. Email is typically appropriate for most healthcare settings because it reaches hiring managers quickly and allows candidates to express appreciation while the conversation remains fresh in the interviewer's memory. Handwritten notes may still be appreciated in some environments, particularly leadership or specialty roles, but timing matters—if postal delivery delays the message significantly, the hiring decision may already be made before the note arrives.

Effective thank-you messages remain concise and specific. A brief expression of appreciation for the opportunity to interview, a reference to one meaningful part of the conversation, and a reaffirmation of interest in the position are usually sufficient. Avoid repeating the entire interview discussion or adding new qualifications that were not previously mentioned. The goal is to reinforce professionalism and interest, not to restate the resume.

For example, a simple structure might include:

- Appreciation for the time spent during the interview

- A short mention of something discussed (unit culture, mentorship programs, patient population, or learning opportunities)

- Confirmation of continued enthusiasm for the role

- A professional closing

Candidates who interviewed with multiple panel members may send individual notes when contact information is available, though one well-crafted message to the hiring manager is often sufficient if additional addresses are not provided. Accuracy in spelling names and titles is essential; small errors can unintentionally create negative impressions.

Thank-you communication also signals follow-through reliability. Nursing roles require consistent documentation, timely communication, and attention to professional detail. Sending a thoughtful follow-up message demonstrates these same habits in the hiring process itself. Recruiters and hiring managers often notice which candidates maintain professional communication after interviews, particularly when multiple applicants present similar qualifications.

Finally, the thank-you message marks a transition point. After sending it, candidates should continue pursuing other applications while waiting for a hiring decision. Maintaining momentum across multiple opportunities prevents unnecessary delays if hiring timelines extend longer than expected, a common occurrence in large healthcare systems where approvals may involve several administrative steps.

A well-written thank-you note does not guarantee an offer, but it reinforces professionalism, strengthens candidate visibility, and demonstrates the communication habits expected in clinical practice. In competitive hiring environments, these small professional signals can quietly support strong interview performance and help keep candidates top of mind as final decisions are made.

Chapter 31
Terms of Care™

Receiving a job offer is an exciting milestone, but the offer itself is only the starting point of a professional agreement. Compensation is only one component of the total employment structure. Schedule design, patient ratios, orientation length, specialty training access, floating expectations, differential pay, benefits eligibility, and tuition assistance programs all contribute to the overall sustainability of the role. Understanding these elements before accepting an offer allows nurses to make decisions that support both immediate career goals and long-term stability.

Base salary typically receives the most attention, yet several additional components often influence actual earnings. Evening, night, weekend, and holiday differentials can significantly increase total compensation depending on the unit schedule. Some organizations also provide specialty pay for high-acuity units, certification bonuses, or clinical ladder incentives tied to professional development activities. Reviewing the complete compensation structure—not just the base hourly rate—helps candidates understand the full financial picture.

Scheduling expectations are equally important. Some units operate primarily on three twelve-hour shifts per week, while others maintain eight-hour or rotating schedules. Candidates should clarify how weekends are assigned, how frequently holiday coverage is required, and whether self-scheduling options are available. Understanding floating policies—whether nurses may be reassigned to other units during staffing shortages—also helps set realistic expectations about daily workflow flexibility.

Orientation and training structures influence early-career success more than many applicants initially realize. Length of orientation, availability of preceptor support, simulation training opportunities, and structured residency programs can significantly affect how smoothly nurses transition into new roles. Asking how competency progression is evaluated and how support is provided during the first months of employment offers valuable insight into how the organization invests in staff development.

Benefits packages also vary widely across healthcare systems. Health insurance eligibility timelines, retirement plan matching, paid time off accrual structures, continuing education reimbursement, and loan repayment assistance programs all contribute to long-term employment value. Reviewing these components carefully ensures that short-term salary comparisons do not overshadow longer-term financial considerations.

Occasionally, organizations include sign-on bonuses tied to employment commitments lasting one to three years.

Candidates should review repayment clauses carefully, understanding how partial employment periods affect repayment obligations if career plans change. Clear understanding at the time of acceptance prevents future surprises.

Professional negotiation does not require aggressive bargaining. Instead, it often involves clarifying details, asking thoughtful questions, and ensuring that expectations are fully understood. Employers generally expect candidates to review offers carefully, and respectful clarification demonstrates professionalism rather than hesitation.

Ultimately, a job offer represents a partnership agreement between the nurse and the organization. Evaluating the complete structure—compensation, schedule, orientation support, professional growth opportunities, and workplace expectations—allows candidates to accept positions with confidence that the role aligns with both personal priorities and long-term career direction.

Chapter 32
Terms of Care™

Accepting a nursing position marks the beginning of a professional chapter that will shape not only clinical skills but also daily routines, lifestyle patterns, and long-term career direction. While job offers often arrive with excitement and urgency, taking time to evaluate the broader structure of the role helps ensure that the position supports both professional growth and personal sustainability.

One of the most important considerations is the **learning environment**. Early-career nurses benefit significantly from structured orientation programs, accessible preceptors, and leadership teams that prioritize mentorship rather than immediate productivity. Units that invest time in teaching often produce stronger long-term clinical confidence, even if the starting pace initially feels slower. Asking how orientation progression is evaluated, how long preceptor support remains available, and what resources exist for ongoing skill development provides valuable insight into how the organization supports new staff.

Staffing patterns also influence daily work experience more than many applicants anticipate. Patient ratios, support staff availability, floating expectations, and the presence of experienced colleagues during shifts affect both workload and stress levels. Observing the unit during interviews—watching how team members communicate, how quickly assistance is available when needed, and how leadership interacts with staff—can reveal cultural patterns that are difficult to identify from job descriptions alone.

Lifestyle compatibility deserves equal attention. Shift scheduling, weekend rotation frequency, commute length, parking availability, and scheduling flexibility all contribute to long-term job satisfaction. Roles that appear ideal clinically may become difficult to sustain if daily logistics create ongoing fatigue or personal life disruption. Evaluating how the position fits into the broader rhythm of life helps prevent early burnout caused by structural misalignment rather than professional difficulty.

Financial considerations also extend beyond starting salary. Tuition reimbursement programs, certification incentives, retirement matching, paid time off accrual, and internal transfer opportunities often influence long-term career mobility. Positions that provide access to specialty training or transition programs may offer greater long-term value even if initial compensation appears similar to competing offers.

Another factor often overlooked is **career mobility within the organization**. Some health systems actively support internal transfers after defined employment periods, allowing nurses to move into specialty areas once foundational experience is gained. Understanding these pathways early helps candidates view the first position as part of a larger career sequence rather than a permanent endpoint.

Finally, trust your early impressions. During interviews, interactions with staff members, tone of communication from leadership, and overall workplace atmosphere often provide subtle signals about unit culture. While no environment is perfect, consistent signs of teamwork, professional respect, and leadership accessibility frequently indicate stronger long-term workplace stability.

Committing to a nursing role is not simply accepting employment; it is selecting the environment where foundational professional habits will develop. Evaluating orientation support, staffing structures, lifestyle compatibility, financial considerations, and growth pathways helps ensure that the first step forward becomes a stable platform for the many career opportunities that nursing offers.

Chapter 33
The 90-Day Pathway™

The first ninety days in a new nursing role shape more than early performance—they establish the habits, relationships, and confidence patterns that often define the first several years of practice. Orientation programs provide the technical framework for learning, but long-term success depends equally on how nurses approach communication, organization, and self-management during this early transition period.

During the first thirty days, the primary focus is learning the operational rhythm of the unit. Every department functions slightly differently, even within the same hospital system. Documentation shortcuts, medication workflows, rounding patterns, escalation procedures, and interdisciplinary communication styles all develop into predictable routines once observed repeatedly. New nurses who prioritize observation, thoughtful questions, and organized note-taking during this phase accelerate their adjustment significantly. Rather than attempting to memorize everything at once, successful learners focus on understanding how the workflow fits together.

The second thirty-day period typically brings increasing independence. Patient assignments may expand gradually, and nurses begin managing more responsibilities with decreasing preceptor oversight. This stage often feels both exciting and stressful as confidence grows alongside accountability. Maintaining structured prioritization habits—starting each shift by reviewing assignments, identifying time-sensitive medications or procedures, and mapping anticipated patient needs—helps prevent small tasks from accumulating into overwhelming workloads. Regular communication with preceptors or charge nurses also ensures that developing concerns are addressed early rather than after problems emerge.

The final thirty days of the initial transition phase emphasize consistency. By this point, many routine tasks begin to feel more natural, allowing attention to shift toward refining clinical judgment, improving efficiency, and strengthening professional relationships across the care team. Nurses who actively seek feedback during this stage often progress more quickly, identifying small performance adjustments that significantly improve workflow confidence.

Across all three phases, relationship-building plays a critical role. Learning the communication preferences of physicians, pharmacists, respiratory therapists, and fellow nurses improves coordination and reduces hesitation during urgent situations. Introducing yourself consistently, asking clarifying questions respectfully, and offering assistance to teammates when possible builds trust that becomes invaluable during busy shifts.

Equally important is self-care and recovery management. Transitioning into new nursing roles can be physically and emotionally demanding, particularly for those adjusting to night shifts, rotating schedules, or high-acuity environments. Establishing consistent sleep routines, maintaining hydration and nutrition during shifts, and allowing adequate recovery time between workdays helps sustain performance during the learning curve. Many early-career burnout experiences occur not because nurses lack clinical ability, but because adjustment stress accumulates without sufficient recovery strategies.

The ninety-day period does not determine whether someone will succeed in nursing, but it strongly influences how confidently that success begins. Approaching this phase with structured learning habits, proactive communication, and realistic expectations allows new nurses to move from orientation dependence toward independent practice with steadily growing confidence. Over time, the routines developed during these first months become the foundation supporting long-term professional growth and clinical effectiveness.

Chapter 34

Confessions of a Healthcare Recruiter™

Quiet Freeze™

Hospitals rarely announce hiring slowdowns publicly, yet internal hiring pauses occur more often than candidates realize. Inside many health systems, staffing approvals are closely tied to financial indicators such as operating margin trends, projected patient census, and liquidity measures like **days cash on hand**—a metric estimating how long the organization could continue operating if incoming revenue suddenly slowed. When leadership becomes cautious about these indicators, hiring activity may not stop outright, but approvals often begin to move more slowly.

Recruiters may continue interviewing candidates, nurse managers may still express strong interest, and job postings may remain active, yet final offer approvals can quietly stall while finance or executive leadership reviews staffing budgets. This temporary approval slowdown is what many recruiters informally call a **Quiet Freeze™**—a period where hiring appears active externally but moves more slowly behind the scenes due to internal financial review cycles. These pauses may last days, weeks, or occasionally longer depending on organizational conditions.

For candidates, the experience can feel confusing. Communication may suddenly decrease, timelines may shift without clear explanation, or a position that seemed ready to move forward may appear to “go silent.” In many cases, the delay is not related to candidate performance but to approval sequencing inside the organization. Understanding this pattern helps applicants interpret hiring delays more accurately and maintain momentum by continuing applications across multiple systems rather than assuming a single delayed opportunity represents rejection.

Healthcare hiring is influenced not only by workforce demand but also by organizational timing. Candidates who remain professionally persistent—following up appropriately, keeping multiple opportunities active, and staying visible to recruiters—are often best positioned to move forward quickly once approval cycles reopen and hiring resumes at full speed.

Chapter 35
Pivot Playbook

One of the greatest advantages of nursing as a profession is the ability to pivot. Unlike many careers where changing specialties requires returning to school entirely, Registered Nurses can transition across a wide range of environments—acute care, outpatient settings, procedural areas, education, case management, informatics, leadership, and community-based roles—often using experience gained in one setting to open doors in another. Understanding how to pivot intentionally allows nurses to adapt their careers as interests, lifestyle priorities, or long-term goals evolve.

Early-career pivots often occur within the first two to three years as nurses discover which environments align most closely with their strengths and preferences. A nurse who begins in medical-surgical care may later transition into ICU, emergency services, or a specialty procedural area after building foundational clinical experience. Others may realize they prefer outpatient settings with more predictable schedules and pursue clinic, ambulatory surgery, or physician-office roles. These early adjustments are common and often represent career exploration rather than instability.

Mid-career pivots frequently reflect lifestyle priorities or evolving professional interests. Nurses seeking reduced physical demands may transition into case management, utilization review, informatics, or patient education roles. Others move toward leadership positions such as charge nurse, clinical educator, or nurse manager, shifting from primarily bedside care to operational coordination and staff development responsibilities. Each pivot builds upon prior clinical knowledge while reshaping daily responsibilities.

Strategic pivoting often involves three coordinated steps: skill alignment, relationship visibility, and targeted credential development. First, nurses identify which competencies from their current role transfer naturally to the desired specialty—assessment skills, patient education, documentation expertise, or procedural familiarity. Second, they increase visibility by networking with managers, educators, or colleagues already working in the target area, expressing interest early rather than waiting for postings to appear. Third, when necessary, they pursue certifications or short-term training programs that demonstrate commitment to the new specialty before formally applying.

Timing also matters. Many specialty units prefer candidates who have demonstrated consistent performance in previous roles, making strong performance evaluations and professional references essential assets during transition attempts. Nurses who maintain professional development portfolios—tracking committee involvement, certifications, continuing education, and leadership participation—often find pivot opportunities easier to access because their readiness is clearly documented.

Importantly, career pivots do not represent abandoning prior experience; they represent expanding professional capability. Skills developed in one nursing environment frequently enhance effectiveness in another. A nurse moving from emergency care to education brings crisis communication experience. A nurse transitioning from ICU to case management contributes deep understanding of complex patient trajectories. Each transition adds perspective rather than resetting professional progress.

Over the course of a nursing career, multiple pivots are not unusual. Interests evolve, life circumstances change, and healthcare delivery models continue to expand into new areas. Nurses who approach these transitions intentionally—building transferable skills, cultivating professional relationships, and preparing for specialty shifts before applying—maintain greater control over their career direction and long-term professional satisfaction.

Chapter 36

Fit Analyzer™

RN Role-Type Fit Mapper — Mini SCRUB*fit*™ Assessment

Becoming a Registered Nurse answers only the first career question. The next—and often more important—question is **what type of nursing environment fits you best**. Nursing spans hundreds of specialties, each with different pace, emotional intensity, decision-making expectations, and lifestyle rhythms. This mini **SCRUB*fit*™** assessment is designed not to determine whether you should be a nurse, but to help identify which **practice environments** are most likely to align with how you naturally work.

Read each statement and rate how strongly it reflects your preferences using the following scale:

1 = Strongly Disagree

2 = Disagree

3 = Slightly Disagree

4 = Neutral

5 = Slightly Agree

6 = Agree

7 = Strongly Agree

Statements

1 I perform well in fast-moving environments where priorities change frequently.

2 I prefer caring for a small number of high-acuity patients rather than many stable patients.

3 I enjoy building long-term relationships with patients and families over time.

4 I feel comfortable working in procedural or technology-focused environments.

5 I prefer predictable daytime schedules whenever possible.

6 I am energized by urgent situations requiring rapid decision-making.

7 I enjoy patient education and coaching individuals through long-term health management.

8 I prefer structured workflows where tasks follow a defined sequence.

9 I am comfortable working independently without immediate team presence.

10 I prefer collaborative team environments with constant interaction.

11 I am interested in roles that allow mobility—moving between locations or visiting patients.

12 I feel most satisfied when I can see measurable recovery progress over time.

13 I am comfortable working with highly technical equipment and monitoring systems.

14 I prefer emotionally steady environments rather than constant crisis exposure.

15 I enjoy roles where organization, coordination, and communication drive outcomes.

Scoring Guidance

Add the numbers from the statements that feel most representative of you and review the patterns below. Most individuals will see strength across multiple categories rather than a single clear outcome.

High scores in 1, 2, 6, 13

Likely alignment: **High-Acuity Acute Care RN**

Examples: ICU, ER, Burn Unit, Critical Care specialties

High scores in 4, 8, 13

Likely alignment: **Procedural / Surgical RN**

Examples: OR, Endoscopy, Outpatient Surgery, Cath Lab

High scores in 3, 7, 12, 14

Likely alignment: **Relationship-Centered RN**

Examples: Oncology, Pediatrics, Rehabilitation, Clinic Nursing

High scores in 5, 9, 11, 15

Likely alignment: **Community / Independent Practice RN**

Examples: Home Health, Case Management, Public Health, Occupational Health

High scores in 10, 15

Likely alignment: **Coordination / Systems-Focused RN**

Examples: Care Coordination, Leadership pathways, Education roles

This tool is not a prediction of your future career. Instead, it functions as an early alignment mirror, helping you notice which work environments may naturally support your strengths and energy patterns. As you continue reading the specialty Day-in-the-Life chapters and hiring guidance sections, revisit your responses. Over time, patterns that initially felt subtle often become clearer, guiding specialty decisions that support both professional effectiveness and long-term career sustainability.

Chapter 37

Alignment Check & Reflection™

By this point in the journey, you have seen multiple versions of nursing life unfold—high-acuity hospital units, outpatient environments, community-based roles, procedural specialties, and independent practice settings. The variety is not accidental. Nursing is one of the few professions where the same license can support dozens of entirely different career experiences, each with its own pace, emotional intensity, technical demands, and lifestyle rhythm. The central question is no longer whether nursing is a strong career option. The question is which version of nursing aligns with how you naturally function.

Alignment does not mean choosing the easiest environment or the highest-paying role. It means identifying the type of work that allows you to sustain performance without chronic depletion. Some nurses thrive in fast-paced emergency settings where rapid decision-making and unpredictable patient flow provide energy rather than stress. Others perform best in structured procedural environments where precision and repetition create a sense of mastery. Still others find the greatest fulfillment in long-term patient relationships, education-focused roles, or community-based care where continuity allows them to witness gradual improvement over time. None of these paths is inherently better than another; they are simply different expressions of the same professional foundation.

Reflection at this stage helps clarify not only interests but also working patterns. Consider how you respond to urgency, how you prefer to structure your day, the environments where your concentration feels strongest, and the type of patient interaction that feels most meaningful. Pay attention to emotional signals as well. The settings that energize you after demanding shifts often indicate stronger long-term fit than those that leave you consistently drained despite adequate skill performance.

Career alignment is also dynamic. The specialty that fits during the early years of practice may not remain the best match later in life as family priorities, lifestyle preferences, or professional interests evolve. Nursing's flexibility allows for these adjustments, enabling clinicians to move between specialties, leadership roles, education pathways, or community-based positions without abandoning the profession itself. Recognizing this flexibility reduces the pressure to identify a single "perfect" specialty early in the career. Instead, think in terms of evolving stages—learning environments, growth environments, and sustainability environments that change as experience accumulates.

Finally, remember that successful nursing careers rarely follow straight lines. Many experienced nurses describe their paths as a series of thoughtful pivots rather than a single predetermined route. Each role contributes skills, perspective, and confidence that shape the next transition. When decisions are guided by alignment rather than momentum alone, those transitions tend to feel intentional rather than reactive.

Take a moment to reflect on what you have learned about yourself while exploring these specialties. Notice which environments captured your curiosity, which responsibilities felt naturally appealing, and which rhythms matched your preferred way of working. These observations are not final answers, but they form the beginning of a decision-making framework that will continue guiding your professional journey long after the first job offer arrives.

Chapter 38

Before You Commit™

Chapter 39
Shortage Indicator

Public discussions often describe nursing as experiencing a nationwide shortage, yet the reality is more complex. Demand for Registered Nurses does not rise or fall uniformly across all specialties, regions, or healthcare settings. Instead, shortages tend to appear in specific geographic areas, high-acuity specialties, and rapidly expanding service lines, while other areas may experience relatively stable staffing conditions. Understanding these patterns helps nurses interpret job-market signals more accurately and position themselves strategically when planning career moves.

High-acuity hospital units frequently demonstrate the most consistent hiring demand. Intensive care, emergency services, perioperative environments, and specialty procedural areas often require additional staffing due to patient complexity, training requirements, and turnover patterns associated with the intensity of the work. Nurses who pursue certifications or specialty training aligned with these areas often find broader employment mobility because these competencies remain in continuous demand across many healthcare systems.

Geographic variation also plays a significant role. Urban academic medical centers, fast-growing suburban regions, and areas experiencing population expansion often maintain higher ongoing hiring activity than locations with stable or declining population trends. Regional workforce demographics—such as retirement rates among experienced nurses—can also create localized demand even when national supply appears stable.

Healthcare delivery changes continue to shift demand as well. Expansion of outpatient surgery centers, telehealth programs, home health services, and chronic disease management initiatives has increased hiring activity outside traditional inpatient hospital settings. Nurses who monitor these industry shifts often identify emerging opportunity areas earlier, positioning themselves for transitions before competition increases.

At times, hiring activity may appear to slow even when demand remains high. Organizational budget reviews, staffing model adjustments, or approval-cycle delays—sometimes experienced internally as temporary hiring pauses—can create short-term fluctuations in posting volume without reflecting long-term workforce needs. Recognizing the difference between temporary hiring slowdowns and sustained workforce demand helps candidates maintain perspective during job searches.

For career planning, the most useful indicator is not whether a generalized "shortage" exists but **where sustained demand intersects with personal interest and long-term**

sustainability. Nurses who align specialty development with areas demonstrating consistent hiring need often maintain greater employment flexibility throughout their careers, particularly during periods of broader economic uncertainty.

Monitoring hiring patterns, certification demand, specialty expansion trends, and regional workforce shifts allows nurses to treat the job market as a set of evolving signals rather than a fixed condition. Over time, this awareness supports more strategic career decisions and helps maintain stability even as healthcare workforce needs continue to change.

Chapter 40

The 101™ — RN Edition

1. What does a typical Registered Nurse shift actually look like?

A typical Registered Nurse shift begins before patient care even starts, usually with a structured handoff report from the previous nurse that outlines patient diagnoses, current conditions, medications, recent changes, and pending tasks. After report, nurses organize their assignments, review orders, check laboratory results, and prioritize care activities that must occur early in the shift, such as time-sensitive medications, procedures, or physician rounds. Throughout the day, patient care involves continuous cycles of assessment, medication administration, documentation, patient education, communication with physicians and interdisciplinary teams, and responding to unexpected changes in patient conditions. Time management becomes one of the most critical skills, as nurses must constantly adjust priorities when emergencies arise or patient needs shift unexpectedly. Breaks may be brief and unpredictable depending on patient acuity, staffing levels, and workflow demands within the unit. By the end of the shift, nurses complete detailed documentation and provide a thorough handoff report to the incoming nurse, ensuring continuity of care before leaving the unit.

2. How long does it usually take to feel confident working independently as a Registered Nurse?

Most nurses begin to feel functional within the first three to six months, but true professional confidence often develops closer to the one- to two-year mark as repeated clinical exposure strengthens judgment and workflow efficiency. Early in practice, new nurses frequently rely on structured checklists, preceptor guidance, and frequent consultation with experienced colleagues while learning how to manage time, prioritize patient needs, and anticipate complications. Confidence grows gradually as common patient scenarios begin to feel familiar and responses to routine changes become more automatic. Exposure to different patient conditions, interdisciplinary teamwork, and increasing responsibility all contribute to a deeper sense of competence. Importantly, confidence does not mean the absence of uncertainty; experienced nurses still ask questions regularly, recognizing that healthcare environments constantly evolve. Over time, consistent experience combined with supportive mentorship typically transforms initial hesitation into steady professional assurance.

3. Which nursing specialties are most competitive to enter as a new graduate?

Specialties such as intensive care, operating room, neonatal intensive care, labor and delivery, and emergency nursing often attract high applicant interest because they offer advanced clinical exposure, strong professional growth potential, and specialized training opportunities. Many hospitals therefore limit entry into these areas through structured residency or fellowship programs that select candidates based on academic performance, clinical rotation evaluations, and demonstrated interest in the specialty. New graduates who complete clinical rotations, internships, or capstone placements within these units frequently gain competitive advantage because hiring managers prefer applicants already familiar with departmental workflows. Geographic location also influences competitiveness, as large academic medical centers often receive far more applications than smaller community hospitals. Candidates who remain flexible about location or initially accept foundational roles such as medical-surgical nursing often find it easier to transition into specialized areas after gaining experience. Strategic career planning therefore often includes building core skills first and pursuing specialty entry through internal transfer opportunities.

4. How important is a nurse residency program for early career success?

Nurse residency programs provide structured transition support that can significantly improve early-career adjustment, particularly in high-acuity hospital environments where workflow complexity can be overwhelming for new graduates. These programs typically include extended orientation periods, classroom learning sessions, simulation training, and mentorship structures that allow nurses to gradually increase independence while maintaining access to experienced guidance. Research consistently shows that residency participation is associated with improved retention, higher job satisfaction, and greater clinical confidence during the first year of practice. In competitive specialties, residency programs often function as the primary entry pathway, making participation essential for nurses seeking early specialization. While nurses can succeed without residency programs, those entering complex hospital settings often benefit from the additional structured support. For many early-career nurses, the residency experience forms the professional foundation that shapes clinical habits and long-term career confidence.

5. What certifications should I plan to pursue during my first few years?

Initial certifications usually depend on the clinical setting, but many nurses begin with foundational credentials such as Basic Life Support (BLS) and Advanced Cardiac Life Support (ACLS), which are commonly required across acute-care environments. As nurses gain experience within specialty areas, pursuing certifications such as CCRN for critical care, CEN for emergency nursing, OCN for oncology, or CNOR for perioperative nursing can enhance both clinical knowledge and professional advancement opportunities. Certification preparation encourages deeper understanding of specialty-specific best practices, often improving clinical decision-making beyond day-to-day experience alone. Many healthcare organizations provide financial incentives or salary differentials for certified nurses, making certification both a professional and financial investment. Timing matters; most specialty certifications require a defined number of clinical practice hours before eligibility. Planning certification goals early allows nurses to track experience requirements and pursue credentials strategically.

6. How often do nurses change specialties during their careers?

Changing specialties is extremely common in nursing and often occurs multiple times across a professional career as interests, lifestyle priorities, and long-term goals evolve. Early-career nurses frequently begin in foundational settings such as medical-surgical units before transitioning into specialty areas once clinical confidence increases. Mid-career transitions may reflect lifestyle changes, such as moving from night-shift hospital roles into outpatient or community-based settings with more predictable schedules. Some nurses pursue leadership, education, informatics, or case-management pathways after years of bedside experience, expanding their influence within healthcare systems. Nursing licensure provides a flexible foundation that allows movement across diverse care environments without restarting education entirely. This flexibility is one of the profession's greatest long-term advantages, enabling career evolution without abandoning clinical expertise.

7. What is the difference between bedside nursing and non-bedside roles?

Bedside nursing focuses primarily on direct patient care, including assessments, medication administration, monitoring clinical changes, patient education, and coordination with interdisciplinary teams. Non-bedside roles, such as case management, informatics, education, quality improvement, or utilization review, shift the focus toward coordination, systems management, data analysis, or program development rather than continuous direct patient interaction. While bedside roles often involve higher physical activity and unpredictable workflows, non-bedside positions may emphasize scheduling predictability, administrative responsibilities, and long-term program outcomes. Both pathways rely on clinical knowledge, but the daily responsibilities and work environments differ significantly. Many nurses transition between bedside and non-bedside roles at different stages of their careers depending on professional goals and lifestyle needs. Understanding these distinctions helps nurses plan career progression more intentionally.

8. How do patient ratios vary across hospital units?

Patient ratios differ widely depending on patient acuity, specialty requirements, and regulatory guidelines within specific states or healthcare systems. Intensive care units may assign one or two patients per nurse due to the complexity of monitoring and treatment demands, while medical-surgical units may involve four to six patients depending on staffing conditions. Procedural and outpatient environments may function differently, focusing more on patient flow rather than fixed ratios. Ratios also fluctuate based on staffing availability, patient census changes, and unexpected admissions. Understanding typical ratio ranges during job interviews helps candidates assess workload expectations more accurately. Staffing structure often plays a central role in both job satisfaction and clinical sustainability.

9. How frequently are nurses required to float to other units?

Floating policies vary across organizations, but many hospitals maintain internal staffing systems that reassign nurses temporarily to units experiencing short-term staffing shortages. Nurses typically float within specialty clusters where they possess baseline competency, such as medical-surgical nurses floating between similar inpatient units. Some organizations provide float-pool positions specifically designed for nurses comfortable working across multiple departments. While floating can increase schedule flexibility and exposure to different specialties, it may also require adapting quickly to unfamiliar workflows. Understanding floating expectations before accepting a position helps nurses prepare for operational realities. Clear orientation and cross-training often make floating experiences smoother and less stressful.

10. What factors influence scheduling flexibility?

Scheduling flexibility is shaped by unit staffing levels, organizational scheduling models, union agreements in some regions, and leadership practices within individual departments. Units using self-scheduling systems often allow nurses to request preferred shifts, though final schedules still depend on staffing needs. High-acuity units or departments experiencing persistent shortages may have fewer scheduling options due to coverage requirements. Seniority systems sometimes influence preferred shift selection, particularly in long-established departments. Communication with scheduling coordinators and early shift-request planning often improves scheduling outcomes. Understanding the scheduling culture of a unit provides valuable insight into long-term lifestyle compatibility.

11. How are night-shift and weekend differentials structured?

Most healthcare systems offer additional hourly compensation for evening, night, weekend, or holiday shifts to incentivize staffing during less desirable hours. Differential amounts vary widely by region, specialty demand, and organizational compensation policies. Nurses working consistent night shifts often experience higher annual earnings due to these additional pay structures. Weekend-only scheduling programs in some facilities offer enhanced differential rates in exchange for consistent weekend availability. Reviewing differential structures carefully during job offers helps candidates understand total earning potential rather than focusing solely on base salary. These supplemental pay components can significantly influence long-term income calculations.

12. How do nurses manage fatigue associated with rotating schedules?

Managing fatigue often requires structured sleep planning, consistent pre- and post-shift routines, and strategic use of rest periods between consecutive workdays. Many nurses develop blackout-curtain sleep environments, scheduled meal timing, and controlled caffeine intake patterns to stabilize sleep cycles despite rotating shifts. Hydration, physical activity, and consistent nutrition during shifts also play important roles in maintaining energy levels. Healthcare organizations increasingly recognize fatigue risks and may implement scheduling policies designed to reduce excessive consecutive work hours. Individual self-care planning remains essential because recovery patterns vary widely among individuals. Long-term sustainability often depends on finding shift patterns that align with personal physiology and lifestyle needs.

13. What is the typical orientation length for new hires?

Orientation length varies by specialty complexity, ranging from several weeks in outpatient settings to several months in high-acuity hospital units such as ICU or emergency departments. Structured orientation typically combines classroom education, simulation training, and supervised clinical assignments gradually increasing in responsibility. Preceptors play a central role in evaluating readiness for independent assignments, adjusting training pace based on individual learning progression. Extended orientation periods often reflect patient acuity rather than organizational inefficiency. Candidates should ask about orientation milestones and competency evaluation processes during interviews. Understanding the support structure helps set realistic expectations for early performance.

14. How does teamwork function during high-acuity situations?

High-acuity clinical environments rely heavily on coordinated teamwork, where nurses, physicians, respiratory therapists, pharmacists, and support staff operate within clearly defined response protocols. During emergencies, communication becomes concise and role-focused, with each team member executing specific responsibilities to stabilize the patient efficiently. Regular simulation training and emergency drills help teams develop familiarity with rapid-response procedures before real situations occur. Effective teamwork reduces decision delays and improves patient safety outcomes. Leadership roles such as charge nurses or response coordinators often guide communication flow during these events. Over time, consistent team interaction builds trust that strengthens emergency response performance.

15. How are clinical decisions escalated when patient conditions change?

Clinical escalation typically follows structured communication pathways designed to ensure rapid response when patient conditions deteriorate. Nurses first assess the patient, implement standing protocols when appropriate, and notify the responsible provider using standardized communication formats such as SBAR (Situation, Background, Assessment, Recommendation). If immediate intervention is required, rapid-response or emergency teams may be activated to provide advanced clinical support. Documentation of assessment findings and communication steps ensures continuity of care and legal clarity. Early escalation is encouraged in modern healthcare environments because timely intervention often prevents more serious complications. Familiarity with escalation protocols becomes one of the most critical safety competencies nurses develop early in practice.

16. What types of continuing education are required to maintain RN licensure?

Continuing education requirements vary by state licensing boards, but most jurisdictions require Registered Nurses to complete a specified number of continuing education hours within each license renewal cycle. These educational activities may include accredited online courses, professional conferences, hospital-based training programs, or specialty certification modules that expand clinical knowledge and professional competencies. Many healthcare employers provide internal education sessions that qualify for continuing education credit, allowing nurses to maintain licensure while developing skills relevant to their workplace. Some states also require training in specific topics such as infection control, patient safety, or opioid-prescribing awareness depending on regulatory priorities. Maintaining organized records of completed continuing education ensures smooth license renewal and avoids administrative delays. Ongoing education supports both regulatory compliance and continuous professional growth throughout a nursing career.

17. How do nurses pursue leadership opportunities?

Leadership pathways often begin informally through participation in unit-based committees, quality-improvement initiatives, or mentorship roles supporting new staff members. Nurses who demonstrate strong organizational skills, effective communication, and reliability during daily assignments are frequently encouraged to pursue charge nurse responsibilities or clinical leadership roles. Formal leadership development programs offered by healthcare systems provide additional preparation in staffing coordination, performance management, and operational decision-making. Advanced education, such as bachelor's or master's degrees in nursing leadership or healthcare administration, may further support advancement into management positions. Networking with nurse managers and expressing interest in leadership opportunities early helps identify available career pathways. Over time, consistent performance combined with leadership involvement often opens doors to supervisory or executive-level nursing roles.

18. What are the most common early-career challenges new nurses face?

New nurses frequently experience challenges related to time management, prioritization, and adapting classroom knowledge to real-world clinical decision-making environments. Learning how to balance multiple patient needs simultaneously while maintaining accurate documentation can initially feel overwhelming. Emotional adjustment also plays a role, as new nurses encounter complex patient situations, difficult family conversations, and the responsibility associated with independent clinical decisions. Supportive preceptors, mentorship relationships, and structured residency programs often ease this transition by providing guidance during the learning curve. Confidence gradually develops as repeated exposure strengthens both technical skills and clinical judgment. Recognizing that early-career discomfort is normal helps nurses remain patient with their own professional development process.

19. How do nurses balance documentation demands with patient care time?

Balancing documentation with direct patient care requires structured workflow habits, including completing charting in real time whenever possible rather than postponing tasks until the end of the shift. Many nurses develop routines such as documenting immediately after medication administration, assessments, or patient education sessions to prevent backlog accumulation. Electronic health record systems increasingly incorporate templates and shortcuts that help streamline documentation while maintaining accuracy. Prioritizing essential charting elements ensures that critical patient information is recorded promptly even during busy periods. Collaboration with colleagues also supports workflow balance, as team members often assist one another when documentation demands temporarily increase. Over time, efficiency improves as nurses become more familiar with both clinical workflows and documentation platforms.

20. What support systems help prevent early burnout?

Support systems that reduce early burnout often include structured mentorship programs, manageable patient ratios, accessible leadership support, and collaborative team cultures that encourage open communication. Peer support networks among fellow nurses provide valuable opportunities to discuss challenging experiences and share coping strategies. Many healthcare organizations now offer employee assistance programs, counseling services, and wellness initiatives designed specifically for healthcare professionals. Maintaining personal routines outside of work—such as consistent sleep patterns, exercise, and social connections—also plays an important role in emotional resilience. Burnout prevention is most effective when both organizational structures and individual self-care practices work together. Early recognition of stress signals allows nurses to seek support before exhaustion becomes overwhelming.

21. How do nurses transition into specialty areas like ICU or OR?

Transitioning into specialty units often involves gaining foundational clinical experience first, followed by application to internal specialty-training or fellowship programs offered by healthcare systems. Many organizations prefer candidates who demonstrate strong performance in general-care environments before advancing into highly technical specialties requiring advanced skill sets. Completing relevant certifications, shadowing experiences, or continuing education courses can strengthen applications for specialty transitions.

Networking with specialty-unit educators or managers also increases visibility when openings become available. Once accepted, nurses typically complete structured orientation programs that include classroom instruction, simulation training, and supervised clinical practice. This staged transition approach helps ensure both patient safety and professional readiness.

22. How does travel nursing work and when is it appropriate to consider?

Travel nursing involves accepting temporary clinical assignments—often lasting several weeks or months—through staffing agencies that place nurses in facilities experiencing staffing shortages. Travel nurses typically receive higher hourly compensation along with housing stipends or relocation assistance, reflecting the temporary nature of assignments. Most agencies require a minimum level of clinical experience, often one to two years within a specialty, before accepting candidates to ensure readiness for fast-paced onboarding. Travel assignments provide opportunities to explore different geographic regions, healthcare systems, and clinical environments while expanding professional experience. However, frequent relocation and rapid orientation expectations may not suit every individual's lifestyle preferences. Careful evaluation of readiness and career goals helps determine the appropriate timing for entering travel nursing roles.

23. What role do professional nursing organizations play in career growth?

Professional nursing organizations provide access to continuing education resources, certification preparation materials, professional networking opportunities, and specialty practice guidelines that support career advancement. Membership often includes reduced conference registration fees, scholarship opportunities, and access to research publications that keep nurses informed about emerging clinical developments. Participation in local or national professional organizations also increases visibility within specialty communities, which can lead to mentorship connections or leadership opportunities. Many nurses discover that involvement in professional groups strengthens both clinical knowledge and professional confidence. Organizational participation demonstrates commitment to professional development and lifelong learning. Over time, these connections often contribute significantly to long-term career growth.

24. How do nurses participate in quality-improvement initiatives?

Quality-improvement initiatives involve structured projects designed to enhance patient safety, improve clinical outcomes, or streamline workflow processes within healthcare systems. Nurses frequently contribute by identifying workflow inefficiencies, collecting patient outcome data, and participating in interdisciplinary committees that develop improvement strategies. Many hospitals encourage staff nurses to propose small-scale improvement projects within their units, allowing frontline clinical insight to guide operational changes. Participation in these initiatives develops analytical skills, leadership experience, and familiarity with healthcare performance metrics. Successful projects may be presented at internal leadership meetings or professional conferences. Quality-improvement involvement often serves as an early pathway into leadership or education roles.

25. How are conflicts with coworkers or providers typically resolved?

Conflict resolution in healthcare environments typically follows structured professional communication practices emphasizing respectful dialogue and patient-centered focus. Nurses are encouraged to address concerns directly with colleagues when appropriate, clarifying misunderstandings before escalation becomes necessary. If issues persist, charge nurses, nurse managers, or human-resources representatives may assist in mediation processes designed to restore effective teamwork. Many organizations provide communication training programs that teach conflict-resolution strategies and collaborative problem-solving techniques. Maintaining professionalism during disagreements helps preserve team cohesion and patient-care continuity. Over time, developing strong communication skills significantly reduces workplace conflict intensity.

26. What malpractice protections are provided by employers?

Most healthcare organizations provide malpractice insurance coverage for employees performing duties within the scope of their assigned roles, offering legal protection if claims arise related to patient care activities. Coverage details vary by employer, including policy limits and circumstances under which protection applies. Some nurses choose to purchase supplemental personal liability insurance to ensure additional coverage beyond employer-provided policies. Understanding policy terms helps nurses clarify their legal protection status in different clinical situations. Employers typically provide information about malpractice coverage during onboarding or orientation sessions. Awareness of these protections supports professional confidence while practicing within established clinical standards.

27. How do nurses prepare for performance evaluations?

Preparation for performance evaluations involves maintaining organized records of professional achievements, continuing education activities, committee participation, and examples of positive patient-care outcomes throughout the year. Reviewing job performance standards in advance allows nurses to align daily practice with organizational expectations. Gathering feedback from preceptors, colleagues, or mentors helps identify both strengths and areas for improvement prior to evaluation meetings. Performance discussions often include goal-setting for the upcoming year, such as pursuing certification, leadership involvement, or skill development initiatives. Entering evaluations prepared with documented accomplishments supports constructive career planning conversations. Consistent preparation transforms evaluations from administrative tasks into meaningful professional development opportunities.

28. What does the clinical ladder system involve?

Clinical ladder programs provide structured pathways for professional advancement that reward nurses for education, certification achievement, leadership participation, and contributions to quality-improvement or research initiatives. Each level within the ladder typically includes defined competency expectations and professional development milestones required for promotion. Advancement often results in compensation increases or recognition within the organization. Participation encourages nurses to expand beyond routine clinical responsibilities while strengthening institutional engagement. Clinical ladder systems also promote retention by providing visible career progression opportunities without requiring movement into management roles. Over time, ladder advancement reflects sustained professional growth and commitment to excellence in practice.

29. How do hospitals measure nursing performance outcomes?

Hospitals evaluate nursing performance using a combination of patient-outcome indicators, safety metrics, documentation accuracy, and patient-satisfaction feedback collected through standardized measurement systems. Metrics such as fall rates, infection rates, medication safety indicators, and readmission patterns often reflect the effectiveness of nursing care coordination. Performance dashboards allow leadership teams to monitor trends and identify improvement opportunities within individual units. Nurses may also receive feedback through peer review systems or competency assessments. These measurement systems aim to support quality improvement rather than solely evaluate individual staff members. Understanding performance indicators helps nurses align daily practice with broader patient-safety goals.

30. How do nurses stay current with evolving clinical guidelines?

Staying current with clinical guidelines requires continuous engagement with professional education, organizational training updates, and specialty association publications that publish evidence-based practice recommendations. Many healthcare systems provide internal education modules whenever clinical protocols change, ensuring staff members receive standardized updates. Specialty certification renewal requirements also encourage periodic review of updated clinical practices. Participation in professional conferences or webinars exposes nurses to emerging research and innovations in patient care. Peer discussions within clinical teams often reinforce guideline updates during daily practice. Maintaining curiosity and commitment to lifelong learning ensures nurses adapt effectively as healthcare standards evolve.

31. What is the difference between charge nurse and nurse manager roles?

Charge nurses typically oversee the operational coordination of a unit during a specific shift, managing patient assignments, assisting with clinical decision escalation, and ensuring staffing coverage meets immediate patient-care needs. Nurse managers, by contrast, hold ongoing administrative responsibility for the entire department, including staffing budgets, hiring decisions, performance evaluations, and long-term operational planning. While charge nurses remain heavily involved in clinical workflow throughout the shift, nurse managers often focus more on leadership, strategic planning, and organizational coordination responsibilities. Many nurses first develop leadership experience by serving as charge nurses before pursuing formal management positions. Understanding the distinction helps clarify career progression pathways within nursing leadership. Both roles contribute significantly to maintaining safe and effective patient-care environments.

32. How often do nurses work mandatory overtime?

Mandatory overtime policies vary widely by organization, state regulations, and staffing conditions within specific specialties. Some healthcare systems restrict mandatory overtime except during declared emergency conditions, while others may require occasional extended shifts during staffing shortages or unexpected patient census increases. Units experiencing chronic staffing challenges may rely more frequently on voluntary overtime incentives rather than mandatory scheduling. Understanding overtime policies during the hiring process helps nurses anticipate scheduling expectations. Many nurses choose positions with predictable scheduling models to maintain work-life balance. Organizational transparency regarding overtime practices often reflects broader workforce-management strategies.

33. How does union representation affect working conditions in some regions?

In regions where nursing unions operate, collective bargaining agreements may establish standardized wage scales, staffing-ratio guidelines, grievance procedures, and scheduling protections that shape working conditions. Union contracts often define overtime policies, benefit structures, and dispute-resolution processes, providing clear frameworks for employment expectations. Some nurses appreciate the structured protections and negotiation support unions provide, while others prefer non-union environments offering more individualized negotiation flexibility. Understanding whether a facility operates under union agreements helps candidates evaluate workplace policies more clearly. Union representation also influences workplace governance structures and leadership communication processes. Familiarity with local labor environments supports informed employment decisions.

34. What are the most common reasons nurses change jobs?

Nurses frequently change jobs due to scheduling preferences, specialty interest transitions, relocation needs, leadership opportunities, or pursuit of improved work-life balance. Workplace culture and staffing conditions also play significant roles in employment decisions, as supportive team environments often influence retention more strongly than compensation alone. Career progression goals, such as moving into advanced practice, education, or leadership roles, may also motivate job transitions. Healthcare system restructuring or service-line expansion sometimes creates new opportunities that attract experienced staff. Job mobility within nursing is relatively common and often reflects career development rather than dissatisfaction alone. Strategic job changes often support long-term professional growth.

35. How do nurses manage emotionally difficult patient situations?

Managing emotionally challenging situations requires a combination of professional communication skills, peer support, and personal coping strategies developed over time. Nurses often rely on interdisciplinary teamwork to navigate complex patient or family conversations, ensuring emotional support responsibilities are shared among care providers. Many healthcare organizations offer debriefing sessions following difficult clinical events to help staff process experiences constructively. Maintaining professional boundaries while expressing empathy helps nurses provide compassionate care without absorbing overwhelming emotional stress. Outside of work, personal support systems and restorative activities contribute to long-term emotional resilience. Over time, experience strengthens the ability to manage emotionally demanding situations while maintaining professional well-being.

36. What resources support mental health for nursing professionals?

Healthcare systems increasingly provide employee assistance programs, counseling services, stress-management workshops, and peer-support networks designed specifically for clinical staff. Professional nursing organizations also offer wellness resources, resilience training, and confidential support services for members experiencing workplace stress. Many hospitals encourage participation in wellness initiatives such as mindfulness training, fitness programs, or structured debriefing sessions following high-intensity clinical events. Personal mental-health practices—including adequate rest, social connection, and reflective downtime—play an equally important role in maintaining psychological well-being. Early utilization of available support resources helps prevent prolonged stress accumulation. Mental-health support is now widely recognized as a critical component of workforce sustainability.

37. How do nurses handle ethical dilemmas in patient care?

Ethical dilemmas often involve complex decisions related to patient autonomy, treatment limitations, end-of-life care, or disagreements among care team members and family preferences. Nurses typically consult with physicians, ethics committees, or leadership teams when complex situations arise, ensuring decisions follow both legal guidelines and professional ethical standards. Many organizations provide formal ethics-consultation services that assist care teams in navigating challenging cases. Clear documentation of patient wishes, advance directives, and care discussions also supports ethical decision-making. Open interdisciplinary communication helps ensure patient-centered care remains the primary focus. Ethical competence develops gradually through experience and professional education.

38. How are shift assignments determined each day?

Shift assignments are generally coordinated by charge nurses or staffing coordinators who balance patient acuity, nurse experience levels, and staffing availability when distributing patient loads. Assignments may change daily depending on admissions, discharges, or clinical complexity fluctuations within the unit. Seniority, specialty certifications, or skill competencies sometimes influence assignment distribution, particularly in high-acuity environments. Effective assignment planning helps ensure both patient safety and equitable workload distribution among staff members. Communication between nurses and leadership allows adjustments when assignments require modification during the shift. Assignment processes are designed to maintain operational efficiency while supporting safe patient care.

39. What is involved in mentoring new graduate nurses?

Mentoring new nurses involves providing guidance on clinical decision-making, time management, professional communication, and adaptation to workplace culture.

Experienced nurses often serve as informal mentors by answering questions, modeling workflow strategies, and offering reassurance during early career challenges. Formal mentorship programs may pair new hires with experienced staff members who provide structured support during the first year of employment. Mentorship relationships help accelerate professional development while strengthening team cohesion. Many experienced nurses view mentoring as both a professional responsibility and an opportunity to contribute to the next generation of clinicians. Effective mentorship significantly improves early-career confidence and retention.

40. How do nurses pursue advanced practice roles such as Nurse Practitioner?

Pursuing advanced practice roles typically requires completing graduate-level education programs such as Master of Science in Nursing (MSN) or Doctor of Nursing Practice (DNP) degrees that provide advanced clinical training. Admission requirements often include active RN licensure, clinical experience, and completion of prerequisite coursework. Many nurses continue working while completing graduate education through part-time or online programs designed for practicing professionals. Specialty selection during graduate training determines future scope of practice, such as family practice, acute care, or psychiatric care. Certification and state licensure processes follow program completion before independent practice begins. Planning educational timelines early helps align career goals with long-term professional advancement.

41. How competitive are graduate nursing programs?

Competitiveness varies by institution reputation, specialty demand, and program capacity, with highly recognized universities often receiving more applications than available seats. Admission committees typically evaluate academic performance, professional experience, recommendation letters, and personal statements demonstrating commitment to advanced practice. Clinical experience in the intended specialty area may strengthen applications significantly. Some programs require entrance examinations or prerequisite coursework before admission eligibility. Early preparation and timely application submission improve acceptance likelihood. Understanding program-specific requirements helps candidates prepare strategically.

42. How long does it take to move into leadership positions?

Leadership advancement timelines vary depending on organizational structure, professional experience, and leadership development involvement. Many nurses begin assuming informal leadership responsibilities such as charge nurse roles within a few years of clinical practice. Formal management positions often require additional leadership training, advanced degrees, or demonstrated operational experience. Participation in committees, quality-improvement initiatives, and mentorship programs often accelerates leadership readiness. Career progression into leadership is rarely immediate but typically evolves through staged professional development. Consistent engagement with leadership opportunities supports long-term advancement.

43. How do nurses maintain work-life balance in high-demand specialties?

Maintaining work-life balance involves careful schedule planning, boundary-setting around extra shifts, and prioritizing rest and personal time outside of work commitments. Many nurses adopt structured recovery routines between shifts to maintain physical and emotional health. Supportive family and social networks also contribute significantly to balance sustainability. Selecting specialties with scheduling models aligned to personal lifestyle preferences can improve long-term satisfaction. Healthcare organizations increasingly emphasize staff wellness initiatives that support balance efforts. Long-term sustainability often depends on both organizational culture and individual self-management strategies.

44. What are the most transferable nursing skills across specialties?

Core skills such as patient assessment, communication, documentation, prioritization, and interdisciplinary coordination transfer effectively across nearly all nursing specialties. Critical-thinking abilities developed through clinical decision-making remain valuable regardless of practice setting. Patient education competencies also translate broadly because teaching responsibilities exist across healthcare environments. Adaptability and teamwork skills help nurses transition more smoothly between departments. Maintaining foundational competencies allows career mobility without restarting professional development. These transferable skills form the backbone of long-term nursing versatility.

45. How do nurses document patient education effectively?

Effective documentation of patient education includes recording the topic discussed, teaching methods used, patient understanding level, and any follow-up instructions provided. Clear documentation ensures continuity of care when other team members review patient records. Many electronic health record systems provide templates that help standardize education documentation processes. Recording patient responses or demonstrated understanding supports quality-of-care evaluation. Accurate documentation also protects legal accountability by confirming that education occurred. Consistent documentation habits strengthen communication across the healthcare team.

46. What happens during hospital accreditation surveys involving nursing staff?

During accreditation surveys conducted by organizations such as The Joint Commission, surveyors evaluate whether hospitals meet established safety, quality, and operational standards, often interacting directly with nursing staff during clinical rounds. Nurses may be asked to explain patient-care procedures, demonstrate knowledge of safety protocols, and show how documentation reflects current patient conditions and treatment plans. Surveyors frequently trace individual patient cases to evaluate how care is coordinated across departments, requiring nurses to discuss medication verification, infection-control practices, and escalation procedures. Preparation for surveys typically includes internal training sessions that review compliance expectations and workflow standards. Although surveys may initially feel stressful, they are designed to reinforce consistent patient-safety practices rather than create punitive environments. Well-prepared teams often find that routine adherence to safety protocols makes survey participation relatively straightforward.

47. How are incident reports handled within healthcare systems?

Incident reports are formal documentation tools used to record events such as patient falls, medication errors, equipment malfunctions, or near-miss situations that could affect patient safety. Once submitted, these reports are reviewed by quality and risk-management teams who analyze contributing factors and identify opportunities for process improvement. The purpose of incident reporting is system learning rather than individual punishment, encouraging staff members to report issues transparently. Confidential review processes help protect staff participation while supporting patient-safety initiatives. Follow-up actions may include workflow adjustments, policy revisions, or additional staff training. Consistent reporting strengthens organizational awareness of safety trends and promotes continuous improvement.

48. What is the role of evidence-based practice in daily nursing decisions?

Evidence-based practice involves integrating current clinical research, professional guidelines, and patient-specific factors into everyday nursing decision-making. Nurses regularly apply evidence-based principles when selecting interventions, educating patients, or evaluating treatment responses. Healthcare systems often provide clinical protocols and guideline summaries to support consistent evidence-based care delivery. Participation in quality-improvement or research initiatives also strengthens nurses' familiarity with current clinical evidence. Applying evidence-based practice improves patient outcomes by aligning care with scientifically validated methods. Continuous learning ensures that clinical decisions remain consistent with evolving healthcare knowledge.

49. How do nurses participate in interdisciplinary rounds?

Interdisciplinary rounds bring together physicians, nurses, therapists, pharmacists, and other healthcare professionals to review patient progress and coordinate treatment plans collaboratively. Nurses contribute bedside observations, patient concerns, response to treatments, and discharge-planning considerations that inform team decision-making. Active participation ensures that nursing assessments influence clinical planning and care adjustments. These rounds also provide opportunities for nurses to clarify orders, discuss patient priorities, and coordinate follow-up interventions. Effective interdisciplinary communication improves both efficiency and patient outcomes. Over time, nurses become central contributors to collaborative care planning processes.

50. What strategies improve communication with difficult patients or families?

Effective communication with challenging patients or families begins with active listening, allowing individuals to express concerns fully before responding. Maintaining calm tone, respectful language, and empathy helps reduce emotional escalation during tense conversations. Providing clear explanations of treatment plans, timelines, and available options often reduces misunderstandings that contribute to conflict. When necessary, involving additional team members such as social workers, patient advocates, or leadership staff can support resolution efforts. Setting professional boundaries while remaining compassionate protects both patient relationships and staff well-being. Consistent communication training strengthens nurses' ability to manage complex interpersonal situations effectively.

51. How do nurses prepare for high-acuity emergencies on the unit?

Preparation for emergencies involves regular participation in simulation training, certification courses such as ACLS or PALS, and familiarity with emergency equipment locations and response protocols. Nurses review rapid-response procedures during orientation and periodic competency evaluations to maintain readiness. Team-based drills help staff practice coordinated communication during critical situations. Knowing escalation pathways and available support teams ensures rapid mobilization when emergencies occur. Maintaining current certifications supports both regulatory compliance and clinical preparedness. Continuous training strengthens confidence in managing urgent patient events.

52. What technologies are most commonly used in modern nursing practice?

Modern nursing practice incorporates electronic health records, automated medication-dispensing systems, patient-monitoring technologies, infusion pumps, telehealth platforms, and clinical decision-support software that assists with medication verification and treatment planning. Nurses interact with these technologies throughout every shift, requiring both technical proficiency and workflow adaptability. Ongoing training ensures staff remain comfortable with system upgrades and new equipment implementation. Technology integration enhances patient-safety monitoring and documentation accuracy. Familiarity with digital systems has become a core competency across healthcare environments. Technological literacy increasingly influences career mobility within specialized settings.

53. How do nurses ensure medication safety during busy shifts?

Medication safety relies on structured verification processes, including patient identification checks, barcode scanning systems, dose verification, and adherence to standardized medication-administration protocols. Nurses often double-check high-risk medications with colleagues to reduce error risk. Organized workflow habits—such as preparing medications in distraction-reduced environments—help maintain accuracy even during busy shifts. Clear documentation of administration times and patient responses ensures continuity of care. Ongoing medication-safety training reinforces best practices. Vigilant adherence to safety protocols significantly reduces adverse medication events.

54. How do staffing shortages affect daily workflow?

Staffing shortages can increase patient ratios, reduce available support staff, and require nurses to manage additional responsibilities during shifts. Workflow adjustments may include prioritizing critical tasks while delegating non-essential duties when possible. Leadership teams often implement contingency staffing plans such as float assignments or temporary staffing support to stabilize operations. Communication among team members becomes especially important during understaffed periods to ensure patient needs remain met. While shortages may temporarily increase workload intensity, strong teamwork often helps maintain safe care delivery. Organizational staffing strategies play a major role in long-term workforce stability.

55. How do nurses advocate for patient safety concerns?

Patient advocacy begins with recognizing potential safety risks and communicating concerns clearly through established escalation channels such as charge nurses, physicians, or rapid-response teams. Nurses document observations thoroughly to ensure clinical concerns are formally recorded. Interdisciplinary collaboration often helps resolve complex safety situations requiring multiple perspectives. Many healthcare organizations encourage a "speak up for safety" culture that supports staff reporting concerns without fear of retaliation. Advocacy efforts may also include participation in safety committees or quality-improvement initiatives. Consistent advocacy strengthens patient-protection systems across healthcare environments.

56. What professional boundaries are important in patient relationships?

Maintaining professional boundaries involves preserving therapeutic relationships focused on patient care while avoiding personal involvement that could compromise objectivity or ethical standards. Nurses provide compassionate support while keeping interactions centered on clinical needs rather than personal relationships. Clear communication of professional roles helps prevent misunderstandings. Organizations provide ethics training that reinforces appropriate boundary practices. Documentation of interactions ensures transparency when complex situations arise. Respecting professional boundaries protects both patient trust and staff professionalism.

57. How do nurses transition from clinical roles to education positions?

Transitioning into education roles often involves gaining clinical experience, pursuing advanced degrees such as MSN or DNP with education focus, and participating in staff-training initiatives within healthcare organizations. Many nurses begin by serving as preceptors or clinical instructors before moving into formal educator positions. Teaching certifications or academic credentials may be required depending on institutional expectations. Educational roles emphasize curriculum development, competency training, and mentorship responsibilities. Clinical experience provides credibility that strengthens teaching effectiveness. Strategic preparation supports successful transition into academic or hospital-education careers.

58. What is involved in becoming a nurse educator?

Becoming a nurse educator typically requires graduate-level education focusing on curriculum development, instructional methods, and educational leadership principles. Educators design training programs, teach clinical skills, and evaluate learner competency across academic or hospital-based settings. Certification in nursing education may enhance professional credentials and employment opportunities. Educators often combine teaching with clinical consultation or research activities. Effective communication and mentorship skills are essential for success in these roles. Nursing education careers support workforce development across healthcare systems.

59. How do nurses enter case management or utilization review roles?

Entry into case management or utilization review often involves developing experience in discharge planning, care coordination, or interdisciplinary communication within clinical settings. Additional certification programs such as Certified Case Manager (CCM) may strengthen professional qualifications. These roles focus on coordinating patient care transitions, evaluating treatment necessity, and supporting efficient healthcare resource utilization. Nurses interested in systems-focused work often pursue these pathways after gaining bedside experience. Organizational training programs sometimes support internal transitions into case-management departments. These roles emphasize coordination rather than continuous bedside care.

60. What types of research opportunities exist for nurses?

Nurses participate in research opportunities through clinical-trial coordination, evidence-based practice projects, academic research partnerships, or hospital-based quality-improvement initiatives that evaluate patient-care outcomes. Some nurses pursue advanced degrees emphasizing research methodology, enabling them to lead independent research studies. Participation in research activities strengthens analytical skills and contributes to advancing healthcare knowledge. Hospitals often maintain research departments that collaborate with clinical staff to collect patient data for approved studies. Publication and conference presentation opportunities may arise from these projects. Research involvement expands professional influence beyond direct patient care.

61. How do nurses prepare for specialty certification exams?

Preparation for specialty certification exams typically involves reviewing official exam blueprints, completing structured review courses, and studying clinical practice guidelines specific to the specialty area. Many nurses join study groups or online preparation communities that provide shared resources and practice-question discussions. Certification organizations often publish recommended reference materials that guide study planning. Consistent study schedules over several months help reinforce both theoretical knowledge and clinical application concepts. Practice examinations allow candidates to identify knowledge gaps before testing. Certification preparation frequently deepens clinical understanding even beyond the exam itself.

62. What are the benefits of obtaining specialty certifications?

Specialty certifications demonstrate advanced clinical competence within a focused area of practice and often enhance professional credibility among peers and leadership teams. Many healthcare organizations provide salary differentials, bonuses, or promotion eligibility advantages for certified nurses. Certification preparation strengthens evidence-based knowledge and improves clinical decision-making confidence. Certified nurses may also gain increased opportunities for leadership roles, committee participation, or specialty program involvement. Professional recognition through certification often supports long-term career advancement. Over time, certifications become visible indicators of professional commitment and expertise.

63. How do nurses manage workplace stress during demanding shifts?

Managing workplace stress often involves developing structured coping strategies such as brief mental-reset breaks, controlled breathing techniques, and prioritization planning that prevents task overload. Supportive communication with coworkers allows team members to assist one another during peak workload periods. Many nurses maintain post-shift routines designed to decompress emotionally and mentally before returning home responsibilities. Organizational wellness programs and peer-support groups also provide resources for stress management. Recognizing early signs of stress helps nurses seek support proactively. Consistent stress-management habits contribute significantly to long-term professional sustainability.

64. How do nurses develop strong prioritization skills?

Prioritization skills develop through experience, mentorship, and repeated exposure to complex patient-care scenarios requiring rapid decision-making. Nurses learn to identify time-sensitive medications, unstable patient indicators, and safety-critical tasks that require immediate attention. Structured communication with charge nurses or experienced colleagues helps refine prioritization decisions during early practice stages. Over time, pattern recognition improves the ability to anticipate patient needs before problems arise. Clinical simulation training often strengthens prioritization learning during orientation programs. Strong prioritization habits become essential for managing multiple patient assignments safely.

65. How do nurses handle unexpected clinical complications?

Handling unexpected complications begins with rapid patient assessment, stabilization actions within nursing scope, and immediate communication with physicians or rapid-response teams when needed. Familiarity with emergency protocols ensures quick initiation of appropriate interventions. Nurses rely heavily on teamwork during these situations, coordinating responsibilities with colleagues to manage complex events effectively. Documentation of clinical changes and interventions ensures continuity of care. Post-event debriefings often provide learning opportunities that strengthen future preparedness. Experience gradually builds confidence in managing unpredictable clinical scenarios.

66. How do nurses improve interdisciplinary communication skills?

Improving interdisciplinary communication involves practicing structured communication methods such as SBAR, participating actively in team rounds, and seeking feedback from colleagues on clarity of information exchange. Observing experienced clinicians during collaborative discussions provides practical communication models. Continuing education programs focused on teamwork and communication also support skill development. Effective communication requires both concise reporting and attentive listening to other team members' perspectives. Regular interaction across disciplines builds professional familiarity that enhances coordination. Strong communication skills significantly improve patient-care outcomes.

67. How do nurses participate in hospital committees?

Hospital committees often include nursing representatives who contribute frontline clinical perspectives to discussions on patient safety, workflow improvement, policy development, or technology implementation. Participation typically begins through volunteer sign-up or manager nomination processes. Committee involvement provides exposure to organizational decision-making structures and leadership opportunities. Nurses often contribute ideas based on daily clinical observations that help improve system efficiency. Committee work also strengthens professional networking within healthcare organizations. Participation supports both career development and institutional improvement initiatives.

68. What is involved in becoming a charge nurse?

Becoming a charge nurse usually requires demonstrated clinical competence, strong communication skills, and the ability to coordinate staffing and workflow decisions during assigned shifts. Many organizations provide leadership-training sessions to prepare nurses for this role. Charge nurses manage patient assignments, assist with clinical escalation decisions, and serve as the primary coordination point between staff and leadership. The role requires balancing administrative responsibilities with continued patient-care involvement. Experience as a charge nurse often serves as preparation for formal leadership positions. Leadership readiness typically develops through both experience and mentorship.

69. How do nurses manage time effectively during busy shifts?

Effective time management involves beginning each shift with structured planning, identifying high-priority tasks, and organizing care activities around medication schedules and patient needs. Many nurses cluster care activities to reduce unnecessary room visits while maintaining patient comfort. Delegation to support staff when appropriate helps distribute workload efficiently. Real-time documentation prevents accumulation of unfinished charting tasks later in the shift. Flexibility remains essential because patient conditions can change rapidly. Over time, refined workflow routines significantly improve shift efficiency.

70. How do nurses prepare for night-shift work?

Preparing for night-shift work often requires gradual sleep-schedule adjustments, creating dark and quiet daytime sleep environments, and maintaining consistent pre-shift routines that signal the body to prepare for nighttime activity. Strategic caffeine use early in the shift and limiting intake later helps maintain alertness without disrupting post-shift sleep. Nutritional planning ensures sustained energy during overnight hours. Many nurses develop consistent exercise and recovery routines that support physical endurance. Communication with family members about daytime sleep needs also helps maintain rest quality. Adapting sleep hygiene practices significantly improves long-term night-shift sustainability.

71. What skills help nurses transition into leadership roles?

Leadership transitions often require development of conflict-resolution skills, delegation abilities, organizational planning competencies, and familiarity with staffing-management systems. Participation in leadership training programs and committee work strengthens these competencies. Mentorship from experienced leaders provides guidance on managing personnel challenges and operational responsibilities. Advanced education in healthcare administration or leadership may further support career progression. Strong communication and emotional intelligence play central roles in effective leadership. Leadership readiness develops gradually through experience and intentional skill-building.

72. How do nurses build professional networks within healthcare?

Professional networking develops through participation in specialty associations, hospital committees, continuing education events, and mentorship relationships with experienced clinicians. Conferences and professional meetings provide opportunities to meet colleagues across healthcare systems. Online professional platforms also facilitate networking connections. Maintaining positive working relationships within the workplace strengthens internal career mobility opportunities. Networking supports knowledge sharing and career advancement awareness. Long-term professional relationships often influence future employment opportunities.

73. How do nurses balance patient advocacy with institutional policies?

Balancing advocacy with institutional policies involves communicating patient concerns clearly through established escalation channels while maintaining adherence to organizational guidelines. Nurses often collaborate with physicians, social workers, and leadership teams to resolve complex situations affecting patient care. Documentation of patient preferences and clinical observations supports advocacy efforts. Ethical consultation services may assist when conflicts arise between patient wishes and institutional policies. Professional advocacy emphasizes respectful communication rather than confrontation. Effective advocacy strengthens patient-centered care while maintaining professional collaboration.

74. How do nurses evaluate potential job offers effectively?

Evaluating job offers involves reviewing compensation, orientation structure, staffing patterns, professional development opportunities, scheduling expectations, and workplace culture indicators observed during interviews. Comparing multiple offers helps identify long-term career growth advantages rather than focusing solely on starting salary. Speaking with current staff members provides valuable insight into daily workflow realities. Considering commute logistics and lifestyle compatibility also influences long-term satisfaction. Understanding organizational stability and advancement opportunities supports strategic decision-making. Thorough evaluation prevents accepting roles that may not support long-term career goals.

75. How do nurses maintain clinical confidence during career transitions?

Maintaining confidence during transitions involves reviewing foundational clinical skills, seeking mentorship within the new specialty, and allowing sufficient adjustment time before expecting full proficiency. Orientation programs provide structured learning opportunities that support skill acquisition. Continuing education courses focused on the new specialty help reinforce knowledge. Open communication with supervisors regarding learning needs ensures appropriate support. Recognizing that adjustment periods are normal reduces unnecessary self-doubt. Confidence typically grows as experience accumulates within the new environment.

76. How do nurses handle workplace conflict professionally?

Handling workplace conflict professionally begins with addressing concerns directly and respectfully with the individuals involved rather than allowing misunderstandings to escalate. Nurses often rely on structured communication techniques that focus on observable behaviors and patient-care impact rather than personal criticism. When conflicts cannot be resolved informally, leadership or human-resources teams may assist in mediation to support constructive resolution. Maintaining professionalism during disagreements protects team cohesion and patient safety. Many organizations provide conflict-resolution training that equips staff with effective communication strategies. Learning to manage conflict constructively becomes an essential leadership skill over time.

77. How do nurses stay current with evolving healthcare regulations?

Nurses remain current with regulatory changes through continuing education courses, professional association updates, employer training sessions, and regulatory board communications. Healthcare systems often provide mandatory education modules that reflect updated compliance requirements. Specialty organizations publish practice updates that help clinicians maintain evidence-aligned care practices. Regular license-renewal processes frequently require documented continuing education hours that reinforce ongoing learning. Staying informed supports both patient safety and professional accountability. Continuous awareness of regulatory changes strengthens clinical practice reliability.

78. What financial planning considerations are important for nurses early in their careers?

Early-career financial planning often includes managing student-loan repayment strategies, building emergency savings, contributing to employer-sponsored retirement plans, and understanding benefits such as tuition reimbursement programs. Shift differentials, overtime opportunities, and specialty incentives may influence income stability during early employment years. Consulting financial-planning resources can help nurses establish sustainable budgeting strategies. Employer benefits packages sometimes include financial counseling services that assist with long-term planning. Strategic financial planning supports career flexibility and long-term stability. Early preparation can significantly improve long-term financial outcomes.

79. How do nurses pursue international or travel nursing opportunities?

Travel and international nursing opportunities typically require a period of clinical experience before agencies consider candidates eligible for temporary assignments. Nurses must ensure licensure compatibility across states or countries, often obtaining additional certifications or regulatory approvals. Travel assignments may offer higher compensation but require adaptability to new clinical environments frequently. Understanding contract terms, housing arrangements, and assignment duration expectations is essential before accepting travel roles. Professional networking and agency research help identify reputable placement organizations. Travel nursing can provide valuable clinical exposure and geographic flexibility.

80. How do nurses support patient families during difficult clinical events?

Supporting families during difficult clinical events involves clear communication, compassionate presence, and coordination with interdisciplinary resources such as chaplaincy, social work, or counseling services. Nurses often serve as primary points of contact who help families understand care updates and treatment decisions. Maintaining calm demeanor and empathy helps reduce anxiety during stressful situations. Providing practical information about next steps or available support services helps families feel less overwhelmed. Respecting cultural and emotional differences ensures individualized support approaches. Consistent family engagement strengthens trust in the care team.

81. How do nurses prepare for performance evaluations?

Preparation for performance evaluations involves documenting accomplishments, continuing education activities, quality-improvement contributions, and professional development milestones throughout the year. Reflecting on both strengths and growth areas allows nurses to participate actively in evaluation discussions. Seeking informal feedback from supervisors before formal evaluations helps identify improvement opportunities early. Many organizations encourage goal-setting conversations that align personal development with departmental priorities. Maintaining a professional portfolio simplifies evaluation preparation. Thoughtful preparation helps ensure evaluations reflect the full scope of professional contributions.

82. How do nurses improve documentation efficiency?

Improving documentation efficiency often involves mastering electronic health record shortcuts, structured templates, and workflow sequencing that integrates charting into patient-care activities rather than postponing it until later. Real-time documentation reduces memory reliance and improves accuracy. Training sessions provided by health systems often teach advanced system navigation skills that save time. Many experienced nurses develop personalized documentation routines that align with their workflow style. Efficiency improves significantly with system familiarity. Strong documentation habits enhance both legal protection and care continuity.

83. How do nurses recognize early signs of burnout?

Early signs of burnout may include persistent fatigue, reduced job satisfaction, emotional detachment, decreased concentration, and feelings of professional exhaustion that extend beyond occasional stressful shifts. Recognizing these indicators early allows nurses to seek support before symptoms intensify. Peer conversations, mentorship discussions, or counseling services may provide early intervention pathways. Adjusting schedules, taking restorative time off, or modifying workload when possible can help restore balance. Many organizations provide burnout-prevention resources that support staff well-being. Early awareness helps maintain long-term career sustainability.

84. How do nurses manage transitions between different shift schedules?

Managing schedule transitions often involves gradually adjusting sleep routines several days before schedule changes, maintaining consistent meal timing, and creating predictable rest environments that support recovery. Limiting abrupt schedule swings when possible helps stabilize circadian rhythms. Many nurses plan personal commitments strategically around shift transitions to maintain energy balance. Hydration, nutrition, and exercise routines also influence adjustment success. Consistent recovery planning improves adaptability. Over time, many nurses develop individualized strategies that minimize disruption during schedule changes.

85. What factors influence long-term career satisfaction in nursing?

Long-term satisfaction often depends on alignment between specialty interests, workplace culture, scheduling preferences, leadership support, and opportunities for professional growth. Nurses who feel supported by their teams and leadership typically report higher engagement levels. Career mobility opportunities also contribute to satisfaction by allowing specialty transitions when interests evolve. Balanced workloads and recognition of contributions further influence retention. Personal purpose and professional meaning derived from patient care remain central motivators. Career satisfaction evolves as professional priorities shift over time.

86. How do nurses participate in disaster-response situations?

Disaster-response participation involves training in emergency preparedness protocols, mass-casualty triage procedures, and coordination with regional emergency-response agencies. Hospitals often conduct simulation drills that prepare staff for large-scale emergency events. Nurses assigned to disaster teams may receive specialized certifications or advanced emergency training. Clear communication systems ensure coordinated response during crisis situations. Participation strengthens community emergency readiness. Disaster preparedness training reinforces the broader public-health role of nursing.

87. How do nurses contribute to infection-prevention programs?

Nurses play central roles in infection-prevention efforts by adhering to hand hygiene protocols, isolation procedures, equipment sterilization standards, and patient-education initiatives related to infection control. Many hospitals involve nursing representatives in infection-prevention committees that review compliance data and improvement strategies. Monitoring patient symptoms and reporting early infection indicators helps reduce transmission risk. Education of patients and families reinforces prevention efforts beyond the hospital setting. Consistent adherence to infection-control protocols significantly improves patient safety outcomes. Infection prevention remains a core nursing responsibility across specialties.

88. How do nurses pursue teaching roles within hospital systems?

Hospital teaching roles often begin with serving as clinical preceptors for new hires or participating in staff-development education programs. Nurses who demonstrate strong teaching skills may transition into formal educator positions within staff-development departments. Continuing education courses in instructional design or adult-learning principles strengthen teaching effectiveness. Many hospitals support certification in nursing education for staff pursuing educator roles. Teaching responsibilities may include competency training, simulation instruction, or policy-implementation education. These roles combine clinical expertise with workforce-development contributions.

89. How do nurses evaluate workplace culture before accepting positions?

Evaluating workplace culture involves observing staff interactions during interviews, asking targeted questions about staffing patterns, mentorship support, turnover rates, and leadership accessibility. Conversations with current employees often provide valuable insight into daily operational realities. Reviewing publicly available employee feedback or professional-network commentary may reveal additional perspectives. Interview follow-up questions about professional development support help assess growth opportunities. Organizational transparency often reflects leadership priorities. Careful culture evaluation helps prevent misalignment between expectations and workplace experience.

90. How do nurses continue developing clinical expertise throughout their careers?

Clinical expertise development occurs through continuing education, specialty certifications, professional conferences, mentorship relationships, and participation in advanced clinical training programs. Exposure to diverse clinical cases strengthens experiential learning over time. Many healthcare systems offer tuition assistance or professional development funding that supports ongoing education. Teaching others often reinforces mastery of clinical concepts. Continuous learning helps nurses adapt to evolving clinical standards and technologies. Long-term expertise develops through sustained professional engagement.

91. How do nurses maintain professional resilience over long careers?

Professional resilience develops through a combination of emotional self-awareness, supportive peer relationships, healthy work-life boundaries, and access to organizational wellness resources. Many experienced nurses cultivate reflective practices that help them process difficult clinical experiences constructively rather than internalizing stress. Maintaining strong personal support systems outside of work also contributes to long-term emotional stability. Periodic career transitions into new specialties or leadership roles may refresh professional engagement when routine fatigue develops. Organizations that prioritize staff recognition and psychological safety often help reinforce resilience among their teams. Over time, resilience becomes a learned professional competency supported by both individual habits and workplace culture.

92. How do nurses prepare for returning to practice after time away?

Returning to practice often involves completing refresher courses, clinical-skills revalidation programs, and reviewing updated regulatory or clinical-practice standards that may have evolved during the absence. Many licensing boards require continuing education completion before reactivation of inactive licenses. Hospitals frequently provide structured re-entry orientation programs that support skill reacquisition. Seeking mentorship during the transition period helps rebuild confidence and clinical familiarity. Reviewing updated technology systems such as electronic health records also supports smoother reintegration. Careful preparation allows returning nurses to resume practice safely and confidently.

93. How do nurses transition into non-clinical healthcare roles?

Transitioning into non-clinical roles often involves leveraging clinical experience to move into areas such as healthcare administration, quality improvement, informatics, case management, or consulting positions. Additional education in leadership, business, or informatics may strengthen candidacy for these roles. Participation in hospital committees or improvement projects can provide relevant experience prior to transition. Networking within interdisciplinary departments often reveals internal career opportunities. Many nurses discover that clinical experience provides valuable system-level perspective highly sought in non-clinical positions. Career flexibility within nursing allows multiple long-term professional pathways.

94. How do nurses protect themselves legally in clinical practice?

Legal protection begins with adherence to professional standards of care, accurate documentation, following established protocols, and seeking clarification when orders appear unclear or unsafe. Many nurses also maintain individual professional liability insurance policies for additional protection beyond employer coverage. Continuing education helps ensure awareness of evolving legal and regulatory expectations. Consulting supervisors or ethics teams when uncertain about clinical decisions supports appropriate action. Professional accountability practices reduce risk exposure significantly. Consistent adherence to standards forms the foundation of legal protection in clinical practice.

95. How do nurses manage career uncertainty or changing professional goals?

Managing career uncertainty often involves periodic self-assessment of professional interests, lifestyle priorities, and long-term aspirations to determine whether adjustments in specialty or role may improve alignment. Continuing education courses or short-term specialty experiences can help explore new areas before committing to full transitions. Mentorship discussions frequently provide insight into potential career directions. Career-planning frameworks help nurses evaluate both immediate and long-term decisions strategically. Recognizing that career paths evolve over time reduces pressure to make permanent early-career decisions. Flexibility supports sustainable long-term career satisfaction.

96. How do nurses evaluate long-term advancement opportunities within organizations?

Evaluating advancement opportunities involves reviewing internal promotion patterns, leadership development programs, tuition-assistance benefits, and specialty training opportunities offered by the organization. Speaking with current staff members about internal mobility experiences provides valuable insight. Observing whether leadership roles are frequently filled internally often indicates organizational commitment to staff development. Understanding performance evaluation and promotion criteria clarifies advancement pathways. Organizations with structured career-ladder systems often provide clearer advancement trajectories. Careful evaluation supports strategic employment decisions.

97. How do nurses mentor colleagues while continuing their own professional growth?

Mentoring colleagues while continuing personal growth involves balancing teaching responsibilities with ongoing education and skill development. Many experienced nurses view mentorship as a collaborative learning process where both mentor and mentee benefit. Participating in mentorship programs also strengthens leadership competencies. Continued engagement in education ensures mentors remain current with clinical standards. Peer teaching opportunities often reinforce professional mastery. Mentorship participation contributes to both workforce development and individual advancement.

98. How do nurses handle major career setbacks such as job loss or specialty dissatisfaction?

Handling career setbacks involves reassessing professional goals, seeking mentorship guidance, updating skills through continuing education, and exploring alternative specialty pathways that may better align with long-term interests. Many nurses discover that setbacks create opportunities to transition into roles more consistent with evolving career priorities. Professional networks often provide leads on new opportunities during transitions. Maintaining professional certifications and licensure readiness supports faster re-entry into employment. Reflective evaluation of previous experiences helps guide more informed future decisions. Career resilience often strengthens after successfully navigating setbacks.

99. How do nurses build long-term professional reputations?

Long-term professional reputations develop through consistent clinical competence, reliability, teamwork, ethical conduct, and willingness to support colleagues during challenging situations. Participation in committees, leadership initiatives, or specialty organizations often increases professional visibility. Positive peer relationships frequently lead to recommendation-based career opportunities. Maintaining professionalism in all workplace interactions reinforces credibility. Continued education and certification achievements further enhance reputation strength. Over time, reputation becomes a significant professional asset influencing career mobility.

100. What habits help nurses sustain long-term career fulfillment?

Habits supporting long-term fulfillment include maintaining strong professional boundaries, prioritizing health and recovery time, pursuing continuing education aligned with personal interests, and periodically reassessing career goals to maintain alignment with evolving life priorities. Many nurses benefit from engaging in professional communities that reinforce purpose and connection. Celebrating small professional achievements helps maintain motivation. Diversifying career experiences over time can prevent stagnation. Intentional reflection on professional impact strengthens sense of meaning. Sustainable fulfillment results from balancing professional dedication with personal well-being.

101. If I'm being completely honest with myself, should I become a Registered Nurse — or would another path fit me better?

Choosing nursing requires more than the desire to help people; it demands sustained comfort with responsibility, unpredictable schedules, emotional intensity, and the reality that clinical decisions often carry immediate consequences for patient outcomes. Some individuals thrive in environments where teamwork, fast-paced problem-solving, and continuous patient interaction define the daily rhythm, while others may find that the constant demand for rapid prioritization and emotional presence gradually drains their energy rather than fuels it. Honest reflection involves asking not only whether you *can* perform the work, but whether the daily environment of healthcare genuinely aligns with how you function best under pressure. Nursing offers extraordinary opportunities for growth, flexibility, and long-term career mobility, yet those benefits are most meaningful when the foundational nature of the work fits the individual performing it. Alignment is less about capability and more about sustainability over decades of professional life.

If the realities of clinical responsibility, evolving technology, interdisciplinary collaboration, and the emotional weight of patient care feel meaningful rather than overwhelming, nursing may provide one of the most dynamic and adaptable careers available in healthcare. However, if the idea of continuous shift-based responsibility, high-acuity decision-making, or physically demanding work consistently feels misaligned with your long-term lifestyle priorities, exploring adjacent healthcare careers may provide equally impactful pathways better suited to your strengths. The goal is not simply entering healthcare, but choosing the role in which you can remain effective, energized, and professionally fulfilled for years to come. The most successful nurses are not those who enter the field by default, but those who recognize that the structure, demands, and purpose of nursing genuinely match how they are wired to work and serve.

Chapter 41

Your SCRUBScript™

Resume Foundations

The modern Registered Nurse resume functions less as a biography and more as a precision document designed to communicate clinical capability, specialty readiness, and measurable impact within seconds of review. Recruiters, hiring managers, and applicant-tracking systems often scan resumes quickly, searching for licensure verification, specialty exposure, certifications, and recent clinical experience that aligns directly with the open role. Because of this, clarity, structure, and keyword alignment matter just as much as experience itself. A well-constructed nursing resume highlights patient-care environments, procedural familiarity, technology systems used, and unit-level responsibilities in a way that immediately signals readiness for the position being pursued. Strong resumes avoid long narrative paragraphs and instead present concise, results-oriented bullet points that demonstrate clinical contributions and workflow competency. The goal is to make it effortless for a reviewer to answer one central question: *Can this nurse step into the role and function safely and effectively?*

Core Resume Structure for Registered Nurses

Every Registered Nurse resume should begin with a clearly visible licensure line placed near the top of the document, ensuring that reviewers immediately confirm active RN credentials and any multistate licensure eligibility. This is followed by a brief professional summary that communicates specialty focus, years of experience, and core clinical strengths relevant to the target role. The clinical experience section should list positions in reverse chronological order, emphasizing patient population served, unit type, average patient load, and major clinical responsibilities. Certifications, specialty training, and continuing education should be grouped in a clearly labeled section to allow rapid scanning by recruiters. Education should follow, listing nursing degree credentials and graduation dates as required by many healthcare credentialing processes. Finally, technology systems, procedural competencies, and specialty equipment experience may be included as a skills section to support keyword recognition within applicant-tracking systems.

Writing Experience That Demonstrates Impact

Hiring teams are not only interested in where a nurse worked, but how the nurse functioned within the unit and what level of responsibility was consistently managed. Instead of listing duties alone, strong resumes describe patient acuity exposure, interdisciplinary coordination responsibilities, and contributions to workflow efficiency or patient-safety initiatives. For example, documenting consistent care for high-acuity patient assignments, participation in rapid-response teams, or involvement in quality-improvement projects demonstrates operational readiness beyond basic task completion. Quantifying experience when possible—such as average patient ratios, procedural frequency, or preceptor responsibilities—helps provide context for workload capacity. Participation in committees, mentorship roles, or specialty training initiatives also signals leadership readiness even early in a career. Impact-focused descriptions allow hiring managers to visualize how the nurse will function within their own department.

Tailoring the Resume to the Target Role

One of the most common mistakes nurses make is submitting the same resume for every application regardless of specialty differences. Tailoring resumes to the target unit by emphasizing relevant clinical exposure significantly increases interview probability. For example, an RN applying to an ICU position should highlight hemodynamic monitoring experience, critical-care certifications, and exposure to ventilator management if applicable, while a nurse pursuing outpatient surgery roles should emphasize procedural preparation, patient education, and recovery-phase care familiarity. Small adjustments in wording that reflect the language used in job postings also improve applicant-tracking system recognition. Tailoring does not require rewriting the entire resume, but it does require adjusting emphasis to reflect the role being pursued. Strategic customization signals professional intentionality and role awareness.

Length, Formatting, and Presentation Standards

Early-career Registered Nurse resumes typically remain one page, while experienced nurses with multiple specialties or leadership experience may extend to two pages when content remains highly relevant. Clean formatting with consistent spacing, readable fonts, and clearly defined section headings improves readability for both human reviewers and automated systems. Avoiding graphics, tables, or complex formatting ensures compatibility with applicant-tracking software used by many healthcare organizations. Consistency in date formatting, credential presentation, and section alignment strengthens professionalism. Even small formatting inconsistencies can create unnecessary distractions during review. Presentation quality communicates attention to detail, an essential clinical competency.

Resume Evolution Across a Nursing Career

Resumes should evolve as clinical exposure expands, certifications are earned, and leadership responsibilities increase. Early resumes often emphasize education, clinical rotations, and residency experiences, while later versions highlight specialty expertise, committee participation, and leadership roles. Updating the resume every six to twelve months ensures that achievements are captured while still recent. Maintaining a "master resume" that includes all experience allows easy customization for specific applications. Career progression is reflected not only in years of experience but also in the increasing complexity of responsibilities listed. A living resume document ensures readiness when unexpected career opportunities arise.

Chapter 42

Intelligent Interviews™

Why Behavioral Interviewing Is Used

Healthcare organizations increasingly rely on behavioral interviewing because past performance patterns often provide the most reliable predictor of future clinical behavior. Rather than asking hypothetical questions, interviewers request real examples that demonstrate how a nurse handled specific clinical, teamwork, or ethical situations. This approach allows hiring teams to evaluate communication style, prioritization ability, accountability, and emotional intelligence—competencies that directly influence patient safety and team performance. Behavioral interviewing also helps distinguish candidates with similar clinical backgrounds by revealing how they think, respond under pressure, and collaborate within interdisciplinary teams. Hospitals invest heavily in onboarding and orientation, so hiring managers aim to select candidates who will adapt successfully to both clinical demands and workplace culture. Understanding this objective helps candidates prepare responses that clearly demonstrate professional judgment and patient-centered thinking.

The Structure Behind Most Behavioral Questions

Most behavioral interview questions follow a consistent framework designed to prompt candidates to describe a real scenario, the actions they took, and the outcomes that resulted. Many organizations train interviewers to listen specifically for decision-making logic, teamwork behaviors, and evidence of reflective learning after challenging situations. Candidates who respond with vague descriptions or hypothetical answers often appear less prepared, even when they possess strong clinical experience. Structured storytelling responses that clearly outline the situation, the challenge involved, the actions taken, and the result achieved allow interviewers to visualize how the nurse functions in real clinical environments. Practicing concise yet complete storytelling responses helps candidates remain confident even when unexpected questions arise. Preparation transforms behavioral interviews from unpredictable experiences into structured professional conversations.

Core Behavioral Themes Hospitals Evaluate

Interviewers frequently evaluate several consistent competency areas, including patient safety awareness, teamwork collaboration, communication effectiveness, accountability, conflict management, and adaptability during workflow disruptions. Many questions are designed to determine how nurses respond when patient conditions deteriorate, when communication breakdowns occur, or when workload demands increase unexpectedly. Interviewers also listen for examples demonstrating professional humility, willingness to seek help when appropriate, and ability to escalate concerns appropriately. Leadership potential may also be assessed even for non-leadership positions by examining how candidates contribute to team stability during stressful situations. Responses that demonstrate calm prioritization, collaborative problem-solving, and patient advocacy tend to resonate strongly with hiring panels. Understanding these evaluation priorities allows candidates to select examples that highlight the competencies organizations value most.

Sample Behavioral Question and Scripted Response Approach

Question: "Tell us about a time when a patient's condition changed unexpectedly. What did you do?"

Scripted Response Framework:

Begin by briefly describing the clinical setting and patient situation, focusing on the key clinical concern rather than unnecessary background detail. Explain the early assessment findings that alerted you to the change and the immediate steps taken to stabilize the patient within your nursing scope. Describe how you communicated with physicians or rapid-response teams, emphasizing clarity and urgency. Conclude by summarizing the patient outcome and any lessons learned that strengthened your clinical practice. Structured responses demonstrate both clinical competence and reflective thinking.

Sample Behavioral Question: Managing Conflict

Question: "Describe a time you had a disagreement with a coworker and how you handled it."

Scripted Response Approach:

Start by outlining the professional context of the disagreement without assigning blame. Explain the steps you took to address the concern respectfully and directly, focusing on patient-care priorities. Describe how communication remained professional and solution-focused rather than emotionally reactive. Share how the situation was resolved or escalated appropriately if necessary. Conclude by explaining what the experience taught you about teamwork and communication.

Sample Behavioral Question: Prioritization Under Pressure

Question: "Tell us about a time when you had multiple urgent responsibilities at once. How did you prioritize?"

Scripted Response Approach:

Begin by explaining the workload scenario and the competing priorities involved. Describe how you assessed patient acuity and identified which interventions required immediate attention. Explain any delegation or teamwork coordination used to ensure all needs were addressed safely. Share the final outcome and how your prioritization protected patient safety. Conclude by describing how experiences like this strengthened your time-management approach.

Preparing a Behavioral Interview Portfolio

One of the most effective preparation strategies involves developing a small portfolio of 8–10 clinical scenarios that demonstrate competencies such as emergency response, teamwork collaboration, patient advocacy, communication challenges, leadership initiative, and conflict resolution. Reviewing these stories before interviews allows candidates to adapt examples quickly to different questions. Many behavioral questions are variations of the same core competency themes, meaning a well-prepared example can be adjusted to fit multiple prompts. Writing brief outlines of these stories improves recall under interview pressure. Preparation also helps responses remain concise rather than overly detailed. Structured preparation significantly increases interview confidence.

Questions Candidates Should Ask Interviewers

Behavioral interviews are also opportunities for candidates to evaluate the organization. Asking questions about mentorship structures, staffing support, professional development opportunities, and leadership accessibility provides valuable insight into workplace culture. Questions about orientation length, continuing education funding, and committee participation opportunities demonstrate professional engagement. Candidates who ask thoughtful operational questions signal long-term career thinking rather than short-term job seeking. Interviewers often remember candidates who engage in meaningful dialogue. Two-way evaluation leads to stronger job alignment.

Final Interview Readiness Strategy

Successful interview preparation combines clinical example preparation, organization research, professional attire readiness, and mental rehearsal of communication pacing. Arriving early, maintaining calm body language, and listening carefully before answering questions improves interview presence significantly. Many candidates benefit from practicing responses aloud rather than silently reviewing notes. Confidence in behavioral storytelling allows the interview to feel conversational rather than interrogative. Interview readiness reflects both preparation and professional composure. The goal is not memorization, but clear demonstration of how you practice nursing in real environments.

Chapter 43
Saying Thank You™

The Power of the Post-Interview Thank-You

In competitive healthcare hiring environments, post-interview thank-you communication remains one of the simplest yet most underused differentiators available to candidates. Hiring teams often interview multiple clinically qualified nurses whose technical skills appear similar on paper, making professionalism, communication follow-through, and perceived team fit important deciding factors. A thoughtful thank-you message reinforces professionalism, confirms continued interest in the role, and provides an opportunity to briefly restate strengths discussed during the interview. It also signals organizational awareness and emotional intelligence, qualities highly valued in patient-care environments where communication reliability matters daily. Recruiters frequently note that candidates who follow up appropriately remain more memorable during final hiring discussions. When executed correctly, the thank-you note is not a formality; it is a strategic reinforcement step in the hiring process.

Timing Guidelines

Thank-you emails are ideally sent within 12–24 hours of the interview while conversations remain fresh in the minds of interviewers. Handwritten notes may also be sent, particularly for leadership or highly competitive specialty roles, though email communication ensures immediate delivery. If multiple interviewers participated, sending individualized notes rather than a single group message demonstrates additional professionalism. Messages should remain concise, professional, and personalized based on interview discussion topics. Excessively long notes are unnecessary and may reduce clarity. Consistency in follow-up communication reinforces professional reliability.

Email Template — Registered Nurse Version

Subject: Thank You — Registered Nurse Interview

Dear [Interviewer Name],

Thank you for taking the time to meet with me regarding the Registered Nurse position. I appreciated the opportunity to learn more about your team, the patient population served, and the collaborative culture within the department. Our discussion reinforced my enthusiasm for the role, particularly the focus on patient-centered care and interdisciplinary teamwork. I am excited about the possibility of contributing my clinical experience and commitment to patient safety to your organization. Thank you again for your time and consideration, and I look forward to the opportunity to work together.

Sincerely,

[Your Name]

Handwritten Note Version

Dear [Interviewer Name],

Thank you for meeting with me to discuss the Registered Nurse opportunity. I appreciated learning more about the team and the department's commitment to high-quality patient care. Our conversation strengthened my interest in joining your organization, and I would be honored to contribute to your clinical team. Thank you again for your time and thoughtful discussion.

Sincerely,

[Your Name]

Short Text-Friendly Follow-Up (When Appropriate)

Hello [Name], thank you again for the opportunity to interview for the RN position. I enjoyed learning more about the team and appreciate your time. I remain very interested in the opportunity and look forward to next steps.

Why This Step Matters More Than Many Candidates Realize

Healthcare hiring often involves multiple approval layers, and final hiring decisions may take days or weeks after interviews conclude. During that time, thoughtful follow-up communication keeps a candidate's name active in the minds of decision-makers without appearing aggressive or intrusive. Hiring managers frequently report that professional follow-up communication reinforces confidence in a candidate's communication reliability—an essential competency in nursing practice. While thank-you notes alone do not secure offers, they often influence final comparisons between similarly qualified candidates. Consistent professional follow-through reflects the same reliability expected in patient-care responsibilities. In highly competitive specialties, small professionalism signals frequently become meaningful decision factors.

Chapter 44

CareerNav™

Finding Roles That Actually Fit

Many Registered Nurse positions are filled long before the broader public ever becomes aware of them. Internal transfers, employee referrals, residency pipelines, and recruiter-managed candidate pools frequently identify candidates early in the hiring cycle, while public job postings often represent the later stages of recruitment visibility rather than the beginning. Understanding this reality shifts job-search strategy from passive application submission toward proactive relationship building, internal networking, and targeted outreach to recruiters and nurse leaders. Monitoring which departments consistently post openings also reveals patterns that may reflect expansion, turnover, or structural staffing challenges. Job boards remain useful, but they represent only one portion of the opportunity landscape. Strategic candidates learn to observe hiring signals rather than relying solely on visible postings.

Effective RN job searching begins with understanding the ecosystem of hiring sources available. Health system career portals provide the most accurate view of internal hiring demand because positions often appear there before aggregating to larger job boards. Professional nursing associations frequently post specialty-specific opportunities not widely advertised elsewhere. Residency program pipelines, continuing education conferences, and specialty certification groups also create informal hiring connections through networking. Maintaining a professional presence on platforms such as LinkedIn allows recruiters to identify candidates even when they are not actively applying. Consistent visibility increases the likelihood of being approached when openings occur.

Patterns in hiring activity can provide important clues about workplace environments. Repeated postings for the same position may indicate growth, internal promotions, or staffing instability depending on the context, making it valuable to research organizational news, expansion announcements, or employee feedback trends. Speaking directly with current employees when possible often provides more accurate insight than relying solely on job descriptions. Understanding whether openings represent opportunity expansion or persistent turnover helps candidates make informed decisions. Strategic job selection focuses not only on obtaining employment but on identifying sustainable work environments aligned with long-term goals. Informed evaluation protects long-term career satisfaction.

Confessions of a Healthcare Recruiter™ — Quiet Freeze™

Inside many healthcare systems, hiring speed is influenced not only by staffing need but also by financial oversight cycles tied to organizational stability metrics such as operating margins, projected patient census, and liquidity indicators like **days cash on hand**, which estimate how long the organization could continue operating if incoming revenue slowed. When leadership initiates internal financial reviews, hiring may not stop entirely, but approval timelines can quietly slow while budgets are reassessed. Recruiters may continue interviewing candidates and managers may express strong interest, yet final offer approvals sometimes pause temporarily while financial authorization processes conclude. Recruiters often refer to these internal approval slowdowns informally as a **Quiet Freeze™**—a period where hiring appears active externally but progresses more slowly behind the scenes. These pauses may last days, weeks, or occasionally longer depending on organizational conditions.

For candidates, a Quiet Freeze™ can feel confusing because communication may decrease temporarily even when interviews were positive. Understanding that these delays frequently reflect approval sequencing rather than candidate performance helps maintain perspective during the hiring process. Continuing to pursue multiple opportunities simultaneously remains the most effective strategy, as approval timelines differ across organizations. Professional follow-up communication after interviews remains appropriate, but patience is often required while internal decisions finalize. Hiring cycles eventually resume full pace once authorization processes reopen. Candidates who remain visible and professionally engaged during these periods are often among the first contacted when approvals move forward again.

Chapter 45

Working With Recruiters

Recruiters play a significant role in Registered Nurse hiring pipelines, particularly within large health systems managing multiple units, specialty openings, and residency cohorts simultaneously. Understanding how recruiters operate allows candidates to work with them strategically rather than passively waiting for opportunities to appear. Recruiters are typically responsible for sourcing candidates, screening qualifications, coordinating interviews, and navigating internal approval processes before offers are extended. Because they often manage dozens of active openings at once, clear communication and responsiveness from candidates significantly improve recruiter engagement. Establishing a professional relationship with a recruiter can lead to visibility for future openings beyond the initial position discussed. Long-term recruiter relationships frequently become recurring career resources as nurses advance.

Candidates benefit from approaching recruiter conversations with preparation similar to interviews, including a clear understanding of specialty interests, scheduling preferences, geographic flexibility, and long-term career goals. Providing concise summaries of experience and certifications allows recruiters to match candidates to appropriate openings more efficiently. Asking informed questions about orientation length, staffing models, and professional development support also demonstrates career seriousness. Recruiters often appreciate candidates who communicate clearly about the types of roles they are willing to consider, as this prevents unnecessary application mismatches. Transparency regarding timeline expectations or competing opportunities helps recruiters coordinate hiring processes more effectively. Strong recruiter communication increases the likelihood of being considered for future openings that may not yet be publicly posted.

It is equally important for candidates to understand recruiter incentives and limitations. Recruiters do not make final hiring decisions; they facilitate the process between candidates and hiring managers while navigating internal approval structures that sometimes extend timelines unexpectedly. Maintaining professional follow-up communication without excessive pressure supports a productive working relationship. Candidates who respond promptly to interview scheduling requests or documentation needs often receive priority attention during competitive hiring cycles. Even when a position is not secured, maintaining positive recruiter relationships often leads to future opportunities when new openings arise. Career progression in healthcare frequently involves multiple recruiter interactions over time.

Professional boundaries also matter when working with recruiters. Candidates should ensure that job details, compensation expectations, and scheduling requirements are clearly confirmed before interviews advance too far in the process. Asking clarifying questions early helps prevent misunderstandings later during offer discussions. Recruiters typically value candidates who communicate respectfully, remain organized, and demonstrate professionalism throughout the hiring process. Building a reputation for reliability and clarity often results in repeat recruiter outreach for future roles. Strategic recruiter engagement transforms hiring from a one-time transaction into an ongoing professional partnership.

Chapter 46

Terms of Care™

Accepting a Registered Nurse position involves more than agreeing to a starting salary. A complete employment offer reflects compensation structure, scheduling expectations, orientation support, benefits, professional development opportunities, and long-term advancement potential. Many early-career nurses focus primarily on hourly rate comparisons without fully evaluating how shift differentials, overtime structures, certification incentives, retirement contributions, and tuition benefits influence total compensation. Understanding the full package allows candidates to make more informed decisions that affect both financial stability and long-term career satisfaction. Offer evaluation should be approached as a structured review process rather than a quick acceptance decision. Careful evaluation prevents unexpected surprises after employment begins.

Compensation in nursing often includes multiple layers beyond base hourly pay. Evening, night, weekend, and holiday differentials can significantly affect annual earnings depending on scheduling patterns. Specialty certifications or advanced clinical competencies sometimes qualify for additional pay incentives. Some organizations offer retention bonuses or sign-on incentives, though these may include employment commitment requirements that candidates should review carefully before accepting. Retirement matching contributions, health insurance benefits, and tuition reimbursement programs may provide long-term financial value exceeding small hourly rate differences. Understanding total compensation rather than base pay alone provides a more accurate comparison between offers.

Scheduling expectations represent another critical component of the offer evaluation process. Candidates should clarify weekend rotation frequency, holiday requirements, floating expectations, and opportunities for self-scheduling if available. Understanding how overtime is offered or assigned helps predict workload stability. Orientation length and transition support programs should also be reviewed, particularly for nurses entering new specialties where extended onboarding may improve long-term success. Units with structured residency or mentorship programs often provide smoother transitions for early-career nurses. Clear scheduling expectations reduce early-career stress and support better long-term retention.

Professional development opportunities within an organization significantly influence long-term career trajectory. Tuition reimbursement programs, certification funding, clinical ladder advancement systems, and leadership-development initiatives all contribute to professional growth potential. Organizations that actively invest in staff education often demonstrate stronger workforce-retention strategies. Asking interviewers about committee participation opportunities, research involvement, or internal promotion patterns helps reveal development pathways. Career mobility within an organization often becomes more valuable over time than initial compensation differences. Strategic career planning includes evaluating growth infrastructure, not only entry-level conditions.

Negotiation within healthcare hiring environments typically focuses less on base salary adjustments and more on scheduling preferences, orientation structure, certification support, relocation assistance, or bonus eligibility when available. Candidates who approach negotiations professionally and respectfully often find organizations willing to accommodate reasonable requests. Preparation for negotiation includes understanding regional compensation benchmarks and clearly identifying personal priorities before discussions begin. Expressing enthusiasm for the role while asking thoughtful clarification questions maintains positive negotiation tone. Negotiation is not confrontation; it is a professional conversation ensuring mutual expectations align. Clear communication during this stage establishes a strong professional foundation for employment.

Final acceptance decisions should only occur after reviewing the complete written offer letter and confirming that all negotiated elements are accurately documented. Verbal agreements should always be reflected in official documentation before final commitment. Taking a short review period before signing allows candidates to consider both immediate benefits and long-term career implications. Consulting mentors or experienced colleagues during the decision process may provide valuable perspective. Thoughtful acceptance decisions reduce early-career job transitions caused by misaligned expectations. Entering a role with clarity supports stronger professional performance from the beginning.

Chapter 47
The 90-Day Pathway™

The first ninety days in a Registered Nurse position represent one of the most important transition periods of an entire nursing career. During this time, nurses are not expected to know everything immediately; instead, the focus centers on safely integrating into workflow systems, understanding unit culture, building team relationships, and gradually increasing clinical independence. Structured orientation programs, preceptor partnerships, and competency checklists are designed specifically to guide this progression. Nurses who approach the first ninety days with intentional learning strategies typically adapt more smoothly and gain confidence faster. Asking questions early is viewed as professionalism, not weakness, particularly in complex clinical environments. The goal of this period is safe growth, not instant mastery.

Days 1–30: Learning the Environment

The first month focuses heavily on orientation logistics, technology familiarity, workflow observation, and initial patient-care responsibilities under close supervision. Nurses learn unit-specific documentation processes, medication-administration systems, emergency response procedures, and communication protocols that vary between organizations. Building relationships with preceptors, charge nurses, and interdisciplinary team members during this period creates early support networks that remain valuable long after orientation ends. Observing experienced staff workflow strategies helps accelerate adaptation to unit pacing. Many nurses find that this phase feels information-heavy, which is expected as new systems and routines are introduced simultaneously. Maintaining organized notes or reference materials during orientation often helps reinforce learning.

Days 31–60: Increasing Responsibility

During the second month, nurses typically begin assuming larger patient assignments while still working closely with preceptors for clinical validation and support. Time-management skills become increasingly important as workflow responsibilities expand. Nurses begin recognizing common patient patterns within their specialty and gain confidence in prioritization decisions. Constructive feedback from preceptors during this phase often accelerates skill refinement. Participation in interdisciplinary rounds becomes more active as nurses contribute clinical observations and care updates. Confidence grows steadily as familiarity with routine scenarios increases.

Days 61–90: Transitioning Toward Independence

By the third month, nurses often function with greater independence while still having access to mentorship and supervisory support when needed. Clinical decision-making becomes more fluid as pattern recognition improves. Nurses typically complete final competency validations and orientation evaluations during this phase, marking the transition into fully independent staffing assignments. Continued learning remains essential, as confidence grows through experience rather than orientation completion alone. Maintaining open communication with leadership about remaining learning needs helps ensure continued development support. Successful completion of the ninety-day transition sets the foundation for long-term professional success.

Habits That Strengthen Early Success

Several consistent habits significantly improve early-career adaptation, including asking clarifying questions early, documenting unfamiliar processes for later review, seeking feedback regularly, and observing how experienced nurses manage complex workflow demands. Developing structured shift-start planning routines also improves organization during early months. Building strong peer relationships provides both clinical support and emotional resilience during adjustment periods. Nurses who approach the early months with curiosity rather than pressure often adapt more comfortably. The first ninety days are designed for growth, not perfection. Intentional learning during this period creates long-term professional confidence.

Chapter 48

Professional Development Roadmap™

Long-term success in nursing rarely occurs by accident; it develops through intentional planning that aligns specialty interests, certification pathways, leadership exposure, and continuing education over time. While early-career nurses often focus primarily on mastering daily clinical responsibilities, gradual planning for future growth helps maintain long-term engagement and career flexibility. Healthcare environments evolve continuously, and nurses who remain proactive about skill development often discover broader professional opportunities. Career progression does not always mean leaving bedside care; it may involve specialization, leadership influence, education roles, or system-level contributions. Understanding potential growth pathways early helps nurses make informed decisions about certifications, graduate education, and committee involvement. Strategic professional development ensures that career movement remains intentional rather than reactive.

Year 1: Foundation Building

The first professional year focuses on strengthening clinical confidence, mastering time management, and developing strong interdisciplinary communication habits. Many nurses begin exploring specialty certification eligibility requirements during this phase to understand future preparation timelines. Participation in mentorship programs or residency cohorts provides structured developmental support. Observing experienced clinicians helps identify long-term specialty interests. Early involvement in unit-based committees or improvement initiatives introduces nurses to organizational leadership processes. Building foundational competence creates the platform for future advancement.

Year 3–5: Specialty Depth

By the third to fifth year of practice, many nurses pursue specialty certifications that formally recognize clinical expertise within specific patient populations or procedural environments. Leadership readiness may begin emerging through charge nurse responsibilities, mentorship of new staff, or committee leadership roles. Continuing education programs during this phase often focus on specialty mastery rather than general clinical orientation. Some nurses begin exploring graduate education pathways aligned with long-term goals such as advanced practice, education, administration, or informatics. Professional networking expands significantly during this stage. Specialty depth often becomes the defining feature of mid-career growth.

Year 5–10: Expansion and Influence

During later career phases, nurses often choose between advanced clinical specialization, formal leadership tracks, academic teaching roles, consulting opportunities, or system-level program development positions. Graduate education completion frequently opens access to broader professional responsibilities. Participation in regional or national professional organizations may increase, providing opportunities for conference speaking, research collaboration, or policy involvement. Mentoring newer nurses becomes a significant professional contribution during this phase. Career direction often becomes highly individualized depending on personal goals and lifestyle priorities. Long-term professional influence typically develops through sustained engagement rather than rapid transitions.

Continuous Career Navigation

Professional development planning should remain flexible because healthcare needs, specialty interests, and personal priorities evolve over time. Periodic career reflection—annually or biannually—helps nurses evaluate whether current roles continue supporting long-term goals. Continuing education funding, certification support, and leadership training availability often influence employment decisions more strongly as careers progress. Career growth does not require constant role changes; meaningful advancement may also occur within the same organization through expanding responsibilities. Intentional planning ensures that professional growth aligns with both clinical passion and lifestyle sustainability. Nursing offers one of the most adaptable long-term career landscapes in healthcare when approached strategically.

Chapter 49

Technology and Innovation™

Technology now shapes nearly every aspect of Registered Nurse practice, from clinical documentation systems and medication-administration verification to patient-monitoring platforms and telehealth integration. Modern nursing environments require both clinical expertise and technological fluency, as nurses interact continuously with electronic systems that support care coordination, safety checks, and interdisciplinary communication. While technology is designed to enhance efficiency and patient safety, adapting to evolving systems requires ongoing learning and workflow adjustment. Nurses who develop strong technology comfort early in their careers often transition more easily across specialties and organizations. Understanding how digital systems influence care delivery helps nurses function more efficiently within complex healthcare environments. Technology literacy has become a core professional competency rather than an optional skill.

Electronic health record systems serve as the central communication hub for most healthcare organizations, allowing nurses to document patient assessments, medication administration, care plans, and interdisciplinary updates in real time. Efficient navigation of these systems improves both productivity and patient-safety tracking. Many organizations provide ongoing training to help staff learn advanced documentation shortcuts that reduce charting time while maintaining compliance. Familiarity with order-verification workflows and alert systems also helps nurses identify potential medication interactions or treatment conflicts more quickly. As health systems continue refining interoperability between departments, documentation accuracy becomes increasingly important. Mastery of EHR workflows significantly influences daily efficiency.

Patient-monitoring technologies continue advancing rapidly, particularly in high-acuity environments such as critical care, step-down units, and specialty procedural areas. Nurses routinely interpret telemetry data, infusion-pump programming, ventilator monitoring information, and early-warning alert systems designed to identify patient deterioration sooner. Understanding how monitoring systems integrate with clinical decision-support tools strengthens early intervention capability. Technology does not replace clinical judgment but enhances the nurse's ability to detect subtle changes earlier. Continuous monitoring environments require both technical familiarity and strong assessment skills working together. The combination of technology and clinical observation forms the foundation of modern patient-safety strategy.

Telehealth expansion has also created new nursing roles focused on remote patient monitoring, virtual triage support, and follow-up care coordination across outpatient settings. Nurses working in telehealth environments often combine clinical assessment skills with digital communication platforms to support patients outside traditional hospital settings. Remote-monitoring programs allow early identification of complications in chronic-care populations, reducing avoidable hospitalizations. As virtual care continues expanding, nurses with telehealth experience may find increasing career opportunities in both hospital-based and community-care systems. Technology-enabled care delivery models are expected to continue growing across healthcare markets. Adaptability to these evolving models supports long-term career flexibility.

Innovation in healthcare technology continues accelerating through artificial intelligence-assisted documentation tools, predictive-analytics monitoring platforms, and automation systems designed to reduce administrative workload. Nurses who remain engaged with continuing education related to digital systems often adapt more easily to these evolving tools. Participation in workflow-improvement initiatives or technology-implementation committees also provides early exposure to new systems. Rather than viewing technological change as disruption, many nurses learn to treat it as an opportunity to improve workflow efficiency and patient-safety outcomes. Comfort with innovation often distinguishes nurses who advance into informatics, leadership, or operational roles. Technology fluency increasingly shapes the future of nursing practice.

Chapter 50

Money Map

Compensation for Registered Nurses extends far beyond the hourly wage printed on the offer letter. While salary provides the baseline, total earnings and long-term financial trajectory are shaped by differentials, specialty opportunities, overtime availability, geographic demand, and professional advancement pathways. Understanding how these elements interact allows nurses to make more informed decisions about both early-career positions and long-term career strategy.

Base pay varies significantly by region, specialty, and experience level. Urban academic medical centers often offer higher starting wages than rural facilities, while high-acuity specialties such as intensive care, emergency services, and procedural environments may include additional pay incentives or specialty differentials. Nurses working evening, night, weekend, or holiday shifts frequently earn supplemental hourly differentials that can meaningfully increase annual income depending on scheduling patterns.

Overtime opportunities also contribute to compensation variability. Some units experience consistent staffing shortages that create regular overtime availability, while others maintain more stable staffing patterns that limit extra-shift opportunities. Nurses who prefer predictable schedules may prioritize stability, while others intentionally select environments where additional shifts allow accelerated income growth during specific career stages.

Certification incentives represent another financial growth pathway. Many organizations offer hourly increases or annual bonuses for specialty certifications such as CCRN, CEN, OCN, or CNOR. These credentials not only improve clinical expertise but also create long-term earning advantages that accumulate across years of practice. Professional ladder programs within health systems may also provide incremental compensation increases tied to leadership participation, committee involvement, research projects, or mentorship responsibilities.

Loan repayment programs, tuition reimbursement benefits, and continuing education support can significantly influence the overall financial value of a position even when base pay appears similar across competing offers. Nurses pursuing advanced degrees or specialty certifications often find that employer-supported education programs reduce long-term financial burden while accelerating career progression.

Geographic mobility also plays a role in income potential. Regions experiencing rapid population growth or persistent workforce shortages frequently offer relocation incentives, sign-on bonuses, or accelerated wage progression structures. Some nurses intentionally relocate early in their careers to build financial momentum before later transitioning to preferred long-term locations.

Finally, long-term earnings in nursing are strongly influenced by career pathway decisions. Advancement into specialty practice areas, leadership roles, education, case management, informatics, advanced practice nursing, or travel nursing can significantly alter compensation trajectories over time. Financial planning therefore becomes less about a single job offer and more about the sequence of roles selected across the first five to ten years of practice.

When viewed strategically, the financial landscape of nursing is not static. Compensation grows through experience, specialty development, certification achievement, and career mobility. Nurses who evaluate opportunities through both immediate earnings and long-term growth potential often build more stable and rewarding financial pathways across their professional careers.

Understanding Total Rewards — The Full Compensation Picture

When evaluating Registered Nurse opportunities, focusing only on hourly wage or annual salary can lead to incomplete financial decisions. Healthcare compensation is structured around a broader framework commonly referred to as **Total Rewards**, which includes both direct pay and the full range of financial and non-financial benefits attached to a position. Two roles offering similar base wages can produce significantly different long-term financial outcomes depending on benefit design, retirement contributions, scheduling flexibility, and education support programs. Nurses who evaluate compensation through a Total Rewards lens often make more strategic career decisions over time.

Direct compensation includes hourly wages, overtime eligibility, shift differentials, weekend premiums, on-call pay, certification incentives, retention bonuses, and performance-based incentives. In many healthcare systems, these supplemental earnings can substantially increase annual income beyond base salary projections. Evening, night, and weekend scheduling patterns frequently carry additional differential structures that meaningfully influence total compensation depending on individual scheduling preferences. Understanding how these differentials are calculated—whether percentage-based or flat hourly additions—helps nurses estimate realistic annual earnings rather than relying solely on advertised starting pay.

Indirect financial benefits often represent an equally important component of long-term compensation. Employer-sponsored retirement contributions, health insurance subsidies, tuition reimbursement programs, student loan repayment assistance, continuing education funding, certification reimbursement, and paid time off policies all carry measurable financial value. Over multiple years of employment, retirement matching programs and education assistance alone can represent tens of thousands of dollars in additional compensation that is not immediately visible in offer letters. Evaluating these benefits carefully allows nurses to compare positions more accurately across organizations.

Work-life structure also plays a financial role within Total Rewards. Scheduling flexibility, self-scheduling systems, compressed workweeks, childcare support programs, and predictable shift patterns can influence both quality of life and financial stability. Roles that provide consistent scheduling may reduce the need for paid childcare adjustments or secondary income scheduling conflicts, indirectly improving overall financial outcomes. Some nurses prioritize higher hourly pay, while others value predictable scheduling structures that support long-term sustainability and reduced burnout risk. Recognizing the financial implications of schedule design ensures that compensation comparisons reflect real-life circumstances.

Finally, career-growth pathways should be considered part of Total Rewards as well. Organizations offering strong clinical ladder programs, leadership-development opportunities, fellowship training, or specialty certification support often accelerate long-term earning potential beyond the first position accepted. Advancement pathways influence compensation trajectory over years, not just starting pay. Nurses who evaluate opportunities based on long-term professional growth frequently build stronger financial stability across the first decade of practice. Viewing compensation through the Total Rewards framework transforms job selection from a short-term wage comparison into a strategic long-term career investment decision.

Chapter 51

Financial Landscape™

Understanding the financial realities of a Registered Nurse career requires looking beyond starting hourly wages to evaluate the full economic structure surrounding the profession. Compensation varies by geographic region, specialty demand, experience level, and organizational type, yet long-term earnings are often influenced just as much by shift differentials, specialty certifications, overtime availability, and career mobility as by base salary alone. Early-career nurses frequently experience steady income growth as clinical experience expands and specialty expertise develops. Strategic financial planning allows nurses to leverage the profession's income stability to build long-term security. Nursing careers often provide predictable earning trajectories compared to many other fields, particularly for individuals willing to pursue specialty certifications or leadership pathways. Financial awareness early in a career significantly improves long-term economic outcomes.

Shift differentials represent one of the most significant compensation variables in nursing, with evening, night, weekend, and holiday shifts often paying additional hourly premiums that can meaningfully increase annual income. Specialty areas such as critical care, operating room, or procedural nursing may also offer incentive pay structures depending on staffing demand. Some organizations provide retention bonuses, relocation assistance, or education reimbursement programs that indirectly increase total compensation value. Understanding how these components interact helps nurses compare offers more accurately. Compensation discussions should always consider the total rewards package rather than hourly rate alone. Long-term earning potential often depends on how strategically nurses navigate these variables.

The Long Payback

Educational debt remains a financial consideration for many nurses entering the profession, particularly those completing BSN or graduate-level programs. Loan repayment planning, employer tuition-reimbursement programs, and federal loan-forgiveness initiatives for eligible service environments can significantly influence financial trajectory over time. Nurses working in underserved areas, public health systems, or nonprofit hospitals may qualify for loan-reduction programs depending on program eligibility criteria. Early exploration of repayment strategies helps reduce long-term financial pressure. Financial counseling services offered through employers or professional organizations can assist with repayment planning. Understanding the long-term impact of loan repayment decisions supports more stable financial planning.

Career mobility also plays a significant role in financial growth. Transitioning into specialty roles, leadership positions, advanced practice pathways, or education careers may increase income potential while also expanding professional influence. Some nurses choose to supplement income through overtime, per-diem assignments, or short-term travel roles during certain career stages. Long-term financial success often reflects career planning decisions rather than initial starting pay alone. Evaluating opportunities for certification pay incentives, leadership stipends, or professional advancement programs helps guide strategic planning. Financial awareness allows nurses to shape income growth intentionally over time.

Finally, retirement planning should begin early, even during the first year of employment. Employer-sponsored retirement plans that include matching contributions provide valuable long-term benefits that compound over decades of employment. Consistent contributions, even at modest levels early in a career, can significantly influence retirement readiness later. Financial literacy resources provided by employers or professional associations often support early planning. Nurses who build strong savings and investment habits early often gain greater career flexibility later in life. Long-term financial stability strengthens overall professional sustainability.

Chapter 52

Side Hustles™ — Income Streams, Flexibility, and Optionality for Registered Nurses

Side hustles in nursing exist for the same reason they exist in life: optionality. Some nurses use side income to accelerate debt payoff, rebuild savings after a hard season, or create breathing room that makes it possible to reduce overtime and protect long-term health. Others use side hustles as a bridge —testing a specialty interest, building a future non-bedside path, or creating flexibility before a move, a family change, or graduate school. The key is to treat side hustles as an alignment decision, not a desperation decision, because poorly chosen extra work can create the same burnout pattern that people were trying to escape in the first place. Nursing offers unusually wide side-hustle options because the skill set is portable, respected, and useful in both clinical and adjacent-clinical environments. The goal is not to chase every opportunity, but to choose income streams that match your energy, schedule, and long-term career direction.

A smart side hustle begins with boundaries. Before picking the hustle, define what you can realistically give without draining your primary role, and be brutally honest about recovery time after shifts. Nurses often underestimate how much "extra" work costs them in sleep, patience, and emotional bandwidth, especially after consecutive twelve-hour shifts. It is also important to understand your employer's policies around moonlighting, conflict-of-interest expectations, and any noncompete language that limits outside work in specific clinical settings. Licensure and malpractice considerations matter as well, particularly if the side hustle involves hands-on patient care, independent health education, or any activity that could be interpreted as clinical decision-making. The safest approach is to keep side hustles clearly within role scope, document your professional boundaries, and avoid anything that blurs clinical authority in informal environments. Optionality only helps if it does not create risk.

Clinical Side Hustles: Extra Shifts Without Extra Chaos

The most common RN side hustle is per-diem or PRN work, often within the same health system or through a local staffing pool. This route is familiar, relatively straightforward to onboard, and can be scheduled selectively when income needs arise. The risk is that per-diem work can quietly become overtime-by-another-name, especially when staffing is tight and extra shifts are consistently available. Nurses who succeed with this path typically choose one additional environment that is either lower intensity than their primary role or structured in a way that feels different enough to prevent emotional fatigue. For example, a high-acuity ICU nurse may find occasional outpatient infusion or procedural recovery shifts more sustainable than adding more critical-care overtime. The strategy is to diversify the stress profile, not multiply it. Side income should reduce financial pressure without increasing clinical burnout.

Travel nursing, local contract roles, and short-term staffing assignments can also function as side-hustle seasons rather than permanent identities. Some nurses choose three- to six-month contract blocks to build savings, then return to stable roles afterward. These assignments often pay more, but they demand adaptability, rapid onboarding, and strong clinical confidence, which can be exhausting if used continuously. If used intentionally, travel or contract work can create short bursts of financial momentum that fund long-term goals like debt payoff, home purchases, or graduate education. The key is to treat these roles like sprints, with planned recovery time afterward. When handled strategically, these temporary roles can become a financial accelerator without becoming a lifestyle trap.

Community and Preventive Care: The "Mobile Health" Option

Community-based side work can be a strong fit for nurses who enjoy education, screening support, and public-facing interaction without the constant crisis rhythm of acute care. Health fairs, vaccine clinics, school-based outreach events, and community wellness programs often hire nurses for weekend or seasonal shifts. This kind of work can feel emotionally lighter for some nurses because the interactions are shorter, the goals are preventive, and the environment is less intense than inpatient care. One creative variation is mobile-health outreach, including community events supported by mobile health buses that bring screenings, education, and basic services into neighborhoods. This work can also expand a nurse's professional network across public health, community organizations, and employer wellness programs. If the nurse's core identity includes teaching and prevention, this side hustle often feels meaningful rather than draining. Optionality is strongest when the side hustle aligns with purpose as well as income.

Education, Training, and Mentoring: Monetizing What You Already Know

Many nurses naturally become informal teachers on their units, and side hustles can formalize that strength. CPR and first-aid instruction, clinical skills tutoring for nursing students, NCLEX support coaching, and simulation lab assisting are common routes that build income without additional bedside burden. Some nurses pick up adjunct teaching roles in local programs once they meet experience requirements, which can create steady supplemental income and professional identity expansion. Another pathway is paid preceptor programs or mentorship initiatives supported by hospitals or academic partnerships, where experienced nurses receive additional compensation for training new staff or students. Education-oriented side hustles often improve the nurse's own clinical mastery by reinforcing foundational knowledge. These roles also build leadership credibility for future educator or management transitions. When aligned correctly, teaching becomes both an income stream and a career-development strategy.

Writing, Content, and Consulting: Turning Clinical Insight Into Influence

Some nurses build side income through writing, education content creation, or consulting work related to patient education, healthcare communication, or workflow improvement. This may include creating patient-friendly education materials, contributing to nursing blogs, consulting on clinical documentation improvement projects, or collaborating with healthcare organizations on training modules. While the internet is full of "quick income" claims, the sustainable version of this path is slower and more professional: build credibility, protect patient privacy, and focus on real value creation rather than viral content. Nurses who succeed here typically choose a niche, such as chronic disease education, perioperative prep teaching, ICU family communication, or nurse onboarding systems. This pathway is not for everyone, but for nurses with strong communication skills and interest in broader impact, it can create long-term optionality. It also offers a future exit ramp from physically demanding bedside roles without leaving healthcare entirely. The key is professionalism, boundaries, and consistency.

What to Avoid: Side Hustles That Create Risk or Burnout

Not all side hustles are equal, and some are bad trades even if the money looks good. Anything that pressures you to practice beyond your scope, make medical recommendations in informal settings, or blur your professional role should be avoided entirely. Be cautious with "wellness influencer" models that encourage unverified claims, aggressive product pushing, or supplement marketing that damages credibility and professional trust. Also be careful with side hustles that require constant availability, unpredictable scheduling, or heavy emotional labor layered on top of an already demanding clinical job. If your nervous system never gets to stand down, the financial gain becomes a long-term cost. The safest hustles preserve your license, protect your health, and strengthen your career rather than undermining it.

Ultimately, side hustles should function like a lever, not a burden. The best side hustles provide income, flexibility, and future options while reinforcing professional strengths and protecting long-term sustainability. Nursing offers more optionality than most careers, and that is a strategic advantage when used thoughtfully. The right hustle can buy you time, reduce stress, fund education, or create a path into a role that fits better long term. The wrong hustle can quietly erode the very stability you were trying to build. Choose optionality with intention, and let the side hustle serve your life—not the other way around.

Chapter 53

Next Moves™

At some point in every Registered Nurse career, the question stops being "Can I do this job?" and becomes "Where should I go from here?" Nursing is one of the few professions where career progression is not linear but modular, allowing clinicians to shift specialties, expand credentials, enter leadership, pursue advanced practice, or transition into adjacent healthcare roles without abandoning the profession entirely. Understanding available next moves early helps nurses avoid feeling trapped in a single specialty when interests or life priorities evolve. Career movement does not always require dramatic change; sometimes the next move is simply choosing the right unit, the right schedule, or the right leadership environment that allows long-term sustainability. Nurses who periodically reassess their direction often maintain stronger engagement across decades of practice. The purpose of this section is to help nurses recognize that staying in the profession does not require staying in the same role forever.

Specialty Transitions

Many nurses begin their careers in medical-surgical or general inpatient environments before transitioning into specialty areas such as intensive care, emergency services, operating room, procedural nursing, oncology, cardiology, or pediatrics. Specialty transitions often require targeted training programs or residency-style onboarding, but prior bedside experience usually strengthens candidacy. Moving into specialty environments can increase both clinical complexity and professional engagement for nurses seeking new challenges. Some specialties also provide more predictable scheduling structures, which may better align with evolving lifestyle needs. Transition planning typically includes obtaining relevant certifications or completing cross-training programs offered within the organization. Specialty mobility remains one of nursing's most powerful career advantages.

Leadership Pathways

Leadership progression often begins with informal roles such as charge nurse assignments, committee participation, or preceptor responsibilities that build operational decision-making experience. Over time, nurses may pursue assistant manager, nurse manager, director, or executive leadership tracks depending on education and career interests. Leadership roles emphasize staffing strategy, quality metrics, team development, and operational planning rather than daily bedside care. Many organizations provide leadership-development programs designed to prepare nurses for these transitions. Advanced degrees in healthcare administration or leadership may support long-term advancement. Leadership pathways allow nurses to influence patient-care systems at broader organizational levels.

Education and Training Roles

Nurses with strong teaching interests often move into educator positions within hospitals, academic programs, simulation labs, or continuing education departments. These roles focus on training new hires, teaching students, or developing competency programs that strengthen workforce readiness. Clinical expertise becomes the foundation for curriculum development and mentorship activities. Many educator roles require graduate-level education focused on teaching methodologies and curriculum design. Teaching positions often provide more predictable schedules compared to bedside roles. Education pathways allow nurses to shape the next generation of clinicians while remaining connected to the profession.

Advanced Practice Nursing

Advanced practice pathways—including Nurse Practitioner, Clinical Nurse Specialist, Nurse Anesthetist, and Nurse Midwife roles—require graduate-level education and specialty certification, but they significantly expand scope of practice and clinical decision-making authority. Nurses considering advanced practice often begin planning several years in advance to meet program prerequisites and experience requirements. Advanced roles may provide increased autonomy, expanded patient-management responsibilities, and new leadership opportunities within clinical teams. These pathways require significant educational investment but offer long-term professional flexibility. Advanced practice represents one of the most recognized long-term growth routes within nursing. Strategic planning helps ensure readiness for these transitions.

Non-Bedside and Hybrid Roles

Not all career growth requires remaining in traditional bedside positions. Nurses frequently transition into roles such as case management, utilization review, informatics, quality improvement, patient safety, clinical documentation improvement, consulting, or healthcare operations positions. These roles leverage clinical knowledge while reducing physical demands associated with bedside work. Hybrid roles combining clinical consultation and administrative responsibilities also exist within many healthcare systems. These pathways often appeal to nurses seeking schedule predictability or system-level influence. Clinical experience remains highly valued even outside direct patient-care environments. Career diversity remains one of nursing's defining strengths.

The Alignment Check

The best next move is rarely defined by salary alone; it is defined by alignment between personal strengths, lifestyle priorities, professional interests, and long-term sustainability. Some nurses thrive in high-intensity clinical environments for decades, while others gradually shift toward education, leadership, or community-based roles as priorities evolve. Periodic reflection—asking whether the current role still fits how you work best—helps prevent burnout-driven career decisions made under stress. Career navigation becomes easier when approached proactively rather than reactively.

Nursing offers a wide map of pathways, but the most successful transitions occur when movement is intentional. The next move is not about leaving nursing; it is about choosing where within nursing you function best.

Chapter 54

Career Longevity Playbook™ — Staying in Nursing for the Long Run

Nursing is one of the few professions that offers both extraordinary career flexibility and extraordinary career demands. Many individuals enter the field with the intention of building lifelong careers, yet the realities of scheduling intensity, emotional exposure, physical workload, and evolving healthcare systems can make long-term sustainability more challenging than new graduates initially expect. Career longevity is rarely accidental; it is typically the result of deliberate professional planning, periodic role adjustments, and intentional strategies that protect both clinical competence and personal well-being over time. Nurses who remain engaged in the profession for decades often do so not because the work is easy, but because they learn how to adapt their roles, schedules, and specialties across different stages of life.

One of the most important principles of career longevity is recognizing that **no single role must last forever**. Early-career nurses frequently believe that leaving a specialty represents a failure or loss of momentum, yet experienced professionals understand that career evolution is both normal and necessary. High-intensity roles such as emergency services, critical care, or procedural environments can provide invaluable clinical experience during certain life stages, while later transitions into outpatient care, education, leadership, case management, informatics, or telehealth roles may offer more sustainable scheduling structures. Viewing nursing as a multi-phase career rather than a single lifelong job allows professionals to remain in the field while adjusting to changing personal priorities, family responsibilities, and physical endurance considerations. Longevity often depends on knowing when to shift roles rather than attempting to remain in the same environment indefinitely.

Physical sustainability also plays a significant role in long-term nursing careers. Repetitive lifting, prolonged standing, and shift-work fatigue can accumulate over years if ergonomic practices and recovery strategies are not prioritized. Nurses who develop habits such as using proper lifting techniques, seeking assistance for heavy transfers, maintaining physical conditioning, and protecting sleep schedules often experience fewer long-term occupational injuries. Healthcare organizations increasingly invest in safe-patient-handling equipment and ergonomic training, yet individual awareness remains equally important. Protecting physical health early in one's career frequently determines the ability to remain clinically active decades later. Longevity planning therefore includes both career strategy and personal health preservation.

Emotional sustainability represents another critical factor. Exposure to suffering, trauma, high patient volumes, and emotionally complex situations can create cumulative stress that gradually erodes professional satisfaction if not addressed intentionally. Nurses who maintain supportive peer relationships, mentorship connections, and reflective practices often navigate emotional demands more effectively than those who attempt to manage stress in isolation. Many experienced professionals describe longevity not as avoiding stress entirely, but as developing coping systems that allow them to process difficult experiences while continuing to find meaning in patient care. Organizations that provide structured debriefing opportunities, peer-support programs, and mental-health resources contribute significantly to workforce retention, yet individual awareness of emotional health remains a personal professional responsibility as well.

Professional growth also contributes strongly to career longevity. Nurses who continue developing new competencies, certifications, or specialty expertise frequently maintain higher levels of engagement and professional motivation over time. Learning new clinical skills, participating in leadership initiatives, contributing to quality-improvement projects, or mentoring newer colleagues can renew professional energy even after many years of practice. Stagnation, rather than workload alone, often contributes to long-term dissatisfaction. Continued learning reminds professionals that the field remains dynamic and that career progression can continue long after initial licensure. Many long-tenured nurses credit ongoing professional development as one of the key factors that kept them engaged across decades of practice.

Financial planning intersects with career longevity as well. Retirement contributions, education investments, specialty certifications, and strategic job transitions all influence long-term financial stability, which in turn affects the ability to make career decisions based on sustainability rather than immediate income pressure. Nurses who approach compensation planning strategically—considering benefits, retirement matching, and long-term advancement opportunities—often gain greater flexibility later in their careers to transition into roles that better match changing lifestyle priorities. Financial stability supports career choice flexibility, which directly influences longevity within the profession.

Finally, one of the most overlooked components of career longevity is **permission to redesign one's career multiple times**. Nursing offers an unusually wide spectrum of practice environments, from bedside care to leadership, education, research, informatics, community health, telehealth, consulting, and policy roles. Professionals who periodically reassess alignment between their role and their evolving personal priorities often remain connected to the profession far longer than those who feel locked into a single career identity. Longevity is not achieved by enduring the same job indefinitely; it is achieved by continuously shaping a career that evolves alongside the professional and personal changes that occur over time. Nurses who embrace this mindset frequently discover that the profession can remain both sustainable and deeply meaningful across the entirety of their working lives.

Chapter 55
Student Success Stories™

Journey 1 — The Career-Changer

At **06:10**, the alarm vibrated across the wooden nightstand before the sun had fully reached the blinds. Elena Martinez, RN, BSN, lay still for a moment, not because she wanted more sleep, but because she still occasionally felt surprised that this was her life now. Ten years earlier, her mornings had begun under fluorescent office lighting, answering corporate emails before finishing her first cup of coffee. Today, her shift in the cardiac step-down unit would begin in less than two hours, and the anticipation she felt wasn't dread—it was focus. Her golden retriever, Milo, padded across the floor and nudged her hand, the daily signal that the day had officially started. She smiled, swung her feet to the floor, and headed toward the kitchen where the coffee maker had already begun its quiet gurgle.

The decision to become a nurse had not come early for Elena. At thirty-two, she had already built what many people considered a stable career in logistics management. The salary was reliable, the hours predictable, and the advancement ladder clearly defined. Yet each year the work felt increasingly detached from the sense of purpose she quietly wanted from her professional life. It wasn't a dramatic moment that changed her direction—no life-altering emergency, no cinematic turning point—just a growing realization that she wanted her daily work to matter in ways spreadsheets never quite delivered. She began researching healthcare careers in the evenings, initially assuming she was "too late" to change directions. The more she learned, however, the more she realized that nursing did not require starting life over; it required starting the next chapter intentionally.

Returning to school was not simple. Elena worked part-time during her accelerated nursing program, balanced coursework with clinical rotations, and spent many evenings wondering whether the transition had been the right decision. The first time she entered a clinical unit as a student, the pace alone felt overwhelming. Machines beeped, call lights flashed, physicians moved quickly between rooms, and experienced nurses seemed to operate with a speed she could barely track. Yet something unexpected happened during those early months: instead of discouragement, she felt engaged. The learning curve was steep, but the work felt tangible. When patients thanked her for small acts—adjusting a pillow, explaining a medication, simply listening—the meaning she had been searching for in her prior career quietly began to take shape.

By **07:05**, Elena had packed her lunch, clipped her badge to her scrub top, and stepped into the early morning air for the drive to the hospital. Traffic was light, the radio low, her mind already organizing the day ahead. Career-changers often bring a different kind of preparation to nursing, shaped by years spent in other industries where communication, organization, and problem-solving were already daily requirements. Elena noticed that many of the workflow-management skills she had developed in logistics transferred directly into patient-care prioritization, helping her manage multiple responsibilities even while still relatively new in practice. Nursing had required new clinical knowledge, but not an entirely new identity; parts of her previous professional life still proved useful in ways she had not expected.

Morning report began at **07:28**, the off-going nurse reviewing each patient's overnight status, medication changes, lab results, and pending care needs. Elena listened carefully, jotting notes in the margin of her patient worksheet while mentally mapping the order in which she would begin rounds. Her assignment included four patients recovering from cardiac procedures, each requiring monitoring, medication coordination, and discharge planning updates. The first hour passed quickly—introductions, assessments, medication checks, communication with the cardiology team—yet the pace felt structured rather than chaotic. Early in her career, she had worried that she might never feel comfortable managing multiple clinical demands simultaneously. Experience, she had learned, gradually converts complexity into familiarity.

Late in the morning, one of her patients, a seventy-six-year-old recovering from a valve repair, grew anxious after receiving new discharge instructions he did not fully understand. Elena pulled a chair closer to the bedside and walked through each instruction slowly, drawing a simple medication schedule on a notepad so he could visualize the routine once he returned home. The interaction lasted only ten minutes, but it reflected something she had not experienced in her previous career: immediate evidence that her work changed someone's day in a meaningful way. Nursing did not eliminate stress, but it replaced abstract productivity metrics with visible human impact. That difference alone had justified the career change many times over.

By **13:15**, the unit settled briefly into a quieter rhythm between admissions. Elena grabbed a quick lunch in the staff break room, laughing with coworkers about the shared reality of eating faster than anyone outside healthcare would consider normal. The camaraderie surprised her when she first entered nursing; teams formed quickly in environments where collaboration was not optional. Experienced nurses shared practical shortcuts, offered quick help when workloads spiked, and provided reassurance during moments that still felt uncertain. Career-changers sometimes worry about entering environments where everyone else seems younger or more experienced, yet Elena found that professionalism and teamwork mattered far more than age. Competence earned respect faster than tenure.

The afternoon moved steadily—coordinating discharge paperwork, assisting with a new admission, updating families by phone, documenting assessments. At **18:55**, she gave evening report to the incoming nurse, ensuring each patient's status and pending needs were clearly communicated. The ritual of handoff once felt intimidating, but now it served as a natural closing marker to the day's work. Walking through the hospital exit doors at **19:20**, she paused briefly in the parking lot, the evening air cooler than when the day began. Some shifts felt heavier than others, but even on difficult days she never experienced the detached feeling that had followed her home from her previous career. The work demanded more energy, yet it returned something in exchange: the sense that her time had mattered.

Driving home, Elena reflected on the fear she once had about changing careers "too late." The reality she discovered was simpler: the right time to move toward aligned work is whenever clarity appears. Nursing had not erased the challenges of working life, but it had replaced quiet dissatisfaction with engagement and purpose. Career-changers rarely describe their transition as easy, yet many describe it as necessary. As she pulled into her driveway, Milo already visible through the front window, she realized the surprise she still felt each morning had not faded—it had simply evolved into gratitude for having chosen a path that finally felt like her own.

Journey 2 — The First-Generation Nurse

At **05:42**, the quiet hum of the apartment's small kitchen fan was the first sound Marcus Hill, RN, BSN, heard as he reached for his phone alarm before it rang. He had learned early that starting the day calmly mattered, especially on shifts where unpredictability was guaranteed. A first-generation college graduate in his family, Marcus still felt a small sense of disbelief each time he clipped his hospital badge onto his scrub top. Growing up, healthcare careers had always seemed like distant possibilities reserved for people with connections or resources his family simply did not have. Nursing had not been an obvious path when he finished high school, but after working several entry-level jobs and watching a close relative navigate a long hospital stay, he began to see the profession differently. What once felt out of reach gradually became a goal he was determined to pursue.

Marcus's route into nursing required persistence more than speed. He began with prerequisite courses at a community college while working evening warehouse shifts to cover tuition expenses. Balancing work and school often meant studying late at night, sometimes reviewing anatomy flashcards during short meal breaks, sometimes listening to recorded lectures during early morning bus rides. Financial pressure made the timeline longer than he initially planned, yet the extended path also strengthened his commitment to finishing. By the time he entered his nursing program, he had already learned how to manage competing responsibilities and long days—skills that later proved essential during clinical rotations. When classmates spoke about the stress of juggling schedules, Marcus often smiled quietly; he had already spent years learning how to do exactly that.

By **06:30**, he stepped outside toward the bus stop, the sky still tinted with the gray-blue light of early morning. Transportation had always been part of his routine, and he used the commute as a mental transition into the clinical environment. Working on a busy urban medical-surgical unit required steady prioritization, quick communication, and the ability to adapt when patient needs changed unexpectedly. Early in his career, Marcus worried that he might struggle to keep pace with more experienced nurses, yet mentorship on the unit made the difference. Senior staff members who remembered their own early struggles often checked in, offering practical advice that no textbook fully captured—how to organize medication passes efficiently, how to anticipate provider questions during rounds, how to maintain calm when multiple call lights activated simultaneously. Supportive teams frequently shape whether early-career nurses build confidence or consider leaving the profession.

Morning report at **06:55** outlined the day's assignment: five patients with varied medical conditions requiring careful monitoring, education planning, and discharge coordination. Marcus reviewed the notes carefully, already mapping the sequence of tasks he would complete during the first two hours of the shift. Time management had become one of his strongest skills, sharpened by years of balancing work, school, and family responsibilities long before becoming a nurse. Nursing demanded clinical knowledge, but it also rewarded discipline, preparation, and consistency—qualities he had built gradually over time. As the shift began, he moved room to room, introducing himself, checking vital signs, and confirming care plans with each patient. Small acts of clarity at the start of the day often prevented larger problems later.

Late in the morning, a patient newly diagnosed with diabetes appeared overwhelmed by the education materials placed at the bedside. Marcus recognized the expression immediately; he had seen the same uncertainty in his own family members when they encountered medical instructions that felt unfamiliar or intimidating. Pulling up a chair, he broke the information into smaller steps, demonstrating how to read glucose-monitor numbers and explaining which daily habits would matter most once the patient returned home. The conversation lasted only a few minutes longer than a standard check-in, but the patient's posture shifted from anxious to relieved by the end. Moments like this reminded Marcus why representation mattered in healthcare—patients often felt more comfortable asking questions when they saw someone who understood their background or communication style. Nursing had become more than employment; it had become a way to create access and reassurance for people who sometimes felt invisible in large medical systems.

By **14:20**, the unit experienced the predictable midday surge of admissions and transport activity. Marcus collaborated with coworkers to prepare rooms, assist with patient transfers, and update documentation before the next wave of medication rounds. The pace rarely slowed entirely, but teamwork made it manageable. During brief breaks, conversations among staff ranged from certification plans to vacation schedules to shared jokes about the realities of twelve-hour shifts. For Marcus, the workplace community carried meaning beyond daily tasks; it represented the professional network that his family had never previously experienced. Becoming a nurse had not only changed his own career trajectory—it had expanded what younger relatives now believed possible for themselves.

Evening handoff at **19:05** brought the familiar closing rhythm of the day. After updating the incoming nurse on each patient's status, Marcus stepped outside into the cooling evening air, shoulders tired but mind steady. The bus ride home offered time to decompress, scrolling briefly through messages from family members who still occasionally asked healthcare questions now that "the nurse" was in the family. Responsibility followed him outside the hospital in small ways, yet he accepted it willingly. Being the first in his family to enter healthcare came with pressure, but it also came with pride. Some journeys into nursing begin with clear guidance;

others begin with curiosity and persistence. As the bus rolled through the evening traffic, Marcus thought about the years it had taken to reach this point and realized something simple: the longer road had still led exactly where he hoped it would.

Journey 3 — The ICU Nurse Who Chose the Long Road

At **05:18**, the low chime of the alarm filled the quiet bedroom before sunrise, and Danielle Carter, RN, BSN, CCRN, reached over to silence it before it could wake the rest of the house. Her husband shifted slightly but remained asleep, while their gray tabby cat stretched across the edge of the bed, entirely uninterested in the day's schedule. Danielle sat up slowly, taking a moment to center herself before the rhythm of the shift began. Intensive care nursing required preparation that was as mental as it was physical; every day held the possibility of rapid clinical change, complex family conversations, and decisions that demanded constant vigilance. She had once imagined becoming an ICU nurse immediately after graduation, but mentors advised her to begin in step-down care first, building assessment confidence before stepping into the highest-acuity environment. At the time, the advice felt like a delay. Years later, she recognized it as the reason she now worked in the ICU with calm confidence instead of constant anxiety.

The kitchen lights came on at **05:32**, coffee brewing while Danielle packed a lunch that would likely be eaten in short bursts between patient rounds. Her path into nursing had not been dramatic; she had always known she wanted a healthcare career, but she also knew she wanted to feel truly prepared before entering critical care. After two years on a cardiac progressive care unit, she applied to the hospital's

ICU transition program, a structured pathway combining additional coursework, mentorship, and simulation-based training. The transition demanded long hours of studying ventilator management, hemodynamic monitoring, and emergency-response protocols, yet the challenge felt purposeful. ICU nursing did not simply require more knowledge; it required the ability to apply that knowledge instantly while coordinating with physicians, respiratory therapists, pharmacists, and fellow nurses under intense conditions. The responsibility was significant, but so was the professional growth.

By **06:10**, Danielle was already on the road, the early morning traffic light and predictable. She preferred arriving early, using the extra minutes to review patient charts before official report began. Preparation created confidence, and confidence created clarity when patient conditions shifted unexpectedly. That morning's assignment included two patients: one recovering from complex cardiac surgery and another requiring close neurological monitoring after a traumatic injury. ICU nurses often manage fewer patients than other units, but the level of monitoring and intervention required for each patient is substantially higher. Small changes in vital signs, lab results, or neurological responses could signal significant clinical developments, making attention to detail critical throughout the shift. Danielle scanned the overnight updates carefully, already anticipating which supplies she might need first.

Morning report at **06:55** was precise, structured, and information-dense, covering ventilator settings, medication titrations, fluid balances, and physician plans for the day. Within minutes of beginning rounds, Danielle adjusted infusion pumps, assessed neurological responses, and coordinated with the respiratory therapist regarding ventilator weaning parameters for one of her patients. ICU nursing often appears intense to observers, yet experienced clinicians learn to operate within a steady rhythm—prioritize, assess, intervene, reassess. Years earlier, Danielle worried she might find the emotional weight overwhelming, but she discovered that strong teamwork distributed the burden. Difficult cases were rarely carried alone; coworkers checked in, physicians discussed options openly, and support systems formed naturally within teams that regularly faced high-acuity care together.

Late in the morning, a patient's family arrived with questions about the recovery timeline following surgery. Danielle walked them through the monitors at the bedside, explaining each reading in clear, non-technical language so they could better understand what they were seeing. ICU nursing frequently includes these moments of translation—turning complex medical information into understandable reassurance for families navigating uncertainty. The conversation lasted longer than a routine update, but Danielle knew the emotional stability of families often improved patient recovery environments as well. Technical skill mattered, yet communication remained one of the most powerful tools ICU nurses carried. Confidence in explaining the situation helped families feel less helpless during difficult days.

By **15:40**, the pace intensified briefly as the care team coordinated imaging transport for one patient while adjusting medications for the other. Danielle worked closely with colleagues, each person managing specific responsibilities while maintaining constant communication. The hours passed quickly, documentation interwoven with assessments, care coordination, and teaching moments for a newly hired nurse shadowing on the unit. Mentoring had become one of her favorite parts of the job; she remembered clearly how intimidating the ICU environment had once seemed, and she made a point of reassuring newer nurses that confidence always came gradually. No one walked into critical care fully prepared—everyone built competence step by step.

Evening handoff at **19:08** brought the familiar sense of transition as Danielle reviewed each patient's status with the incoming nurse, ensuring that subtle trends from the day were clearly communicated. Walking out to the parking garage at **19:35**, she felt the usual physical fatigue that followed a twelve-hour shift, yet mentally she remained steady. ICU nursing demanded sustained focus, but it also provided a level of professional fulfillment she had not found elsewhere. The long road she had taken—step-down first, ICU later—had once felt like a delay. Now she understood it differently: it had been preparation. As she started the car and merged into the evening traffic, she thought briefly about the younger version of herself eager to move faster and smiled at the realization that sometimes the longer route is the one that makes the destination sustainable.

Journey 4 — The Single Parent Who Refused to Quit

At **04:58**, the alarm lit the small bedroom with a soft blue glow, and Tanya Brooks, RN, BSN, reached across the nightstand before it could ring loudly enough to wake her eight-year-old son in the next room. Morning routines in her household followed a precise rhythm because precision created calm, and calm made long days manageable. Coffee brewed while she packed a lunch, checked the school backpack waiting by the door, and glanced once more at the weekly calendar taped to the refrigerator—shift times, school pickup arrangements, and the occasional reminder to herself that this life, busy as it was, had once seemed nearly impossible to reach. Years earlier, nursing school had felt like an unrealistic dream for a single parent balancing work, childcare, and financial pressure. The path had been longer than she originally imagined, but she had learned something along the way: progress did not require perfect conditions; it required persistence.

Tanya began her journey into healthcare working as a patient care technician, taking night shifts that allowed her to attend classes during the day while family members helped with childcare. Many semesters stretched longer than planned, not because she lacked motivation, but because life required adjustments—illnesses, unexpected expenses, scheduling conflicts that forced course rescheduling. At times, the extended timeline felt discouraging, yet each completed prerequisite course built momentum that gradually replaced doubt with confidence. By the time she entered her nursing program, she had already developed a resilience that would later serve her well during the most demanding clinical rotations. Nursing education tested academic knowledge, but it also quietly tested endurance, organization, and emotional strength. Tanya discovered she possessed more of each than she once believed.

By **05:45**, she woke her son gently, helping him prepare for school while finishing her own preparations for the day. The commute to the hospital took twenty-five minutes, just long enough for her to mentally organize the priorities waiting ahead. Working on a high-volume medical-surgical floor required flexibility, efficient communication, and the ability to shift plans quickly when admissions increased or patient conditions changed. Early in her career, she worried constantly about making mistakes, double-checking every medication and reviewing every order with extra caution. Over time, experience replaced constant anxiety with steady confidence, though the responsibility never felt routine. Nursing demanded attentiveness every day, regardless of how many shifts had come before it.

Morning report at **06:52** outlined a full assignment: five patients with varied diagnoses, discharge planning underway for two, and a pending admission expected before midday. Tanya noted key details carefully, then began the familiar sequence—introductions, safety checks, medication preparation, and coordination with physicians rounding on the unit. One of her patients, a middle-aged man recovering from surgery, appeared visibly discouraged about the expected recovery timeline. Tanya paused to explain the progression step by step, emphasizing realistic milestones rather than distant outcomes. These conversations often required patience, but she understood something from personal experience: progress feels easier when people understand what comes next. Nursing was not only about interventions; it was also about helping patients navigate uncertainty.

Midday brought the predictable rush of transport calls, lab draws, and discharge paperwork, yet teamwork kept the pace manageable. Coworkers assisted one another without needing to be asked, a culture Tanya had come to rely on during especially busy shifts. In quieter moments, she sometimes thought back to the years when returning to school seemed nearly impossible financially and logistically. Now, standing in the center of the unit coordinating care plans, she recognized how dramatically persistence could change a life trajectory. Her son occasionally told friends, "My mom's a nurse," with the kind of pride that made every difficult semester worthwhile. The profession had not only provided career stability—it had reshaped what her family believed was possible.

By **19:18**, after evening handoff, Tanya stepped outside into the cooling air, shoulders tired but mind steady. The drive home included a quick stop to pick up her son from a neighbor who helped with after-school care on shift days, followed by dinner conversations about homework, soccer practice, and the ordinary details that formed the center of their shared routine. Nursing schedules were demanding, yet the condensed workweek also created full days off that she reserved intentionally for family time. Balance did not appear automatically; it required planning, coordination, and occasional sacrifice. Still, as she tucked her son into bed later that night, she felt a quiet sense of accomplishment that extended beyond the hospital walls. Some journeys into nursing begin with opportunity; others begin with determination. Tanya's had begun with both necessity and hope—and she had refused to let either go unfinished.

Journey 5 — The Military Medic Transition

At **05:36**, the steady vibration of the phone alarm cut through the quiet apartment, and Jason Walker, RN, BSN, sat up almost immediately, years of military routine still shaping how he started each morning. Even after several years in civilian healthcare, he preferred rising early, giving himself time to prepare mentally before the pace of the hospital day began. A framed photograph of his former unit rested on the dresser across the room, a reminder of the path that had first introduced him to emergency medicine long before he ever considered becoming a Registered Nurse. During his service, Jason had worked as a combat medic, gaining experience responding to trauma, stabilizing injuries, and making rapid decisions under pressure. When he returned to civilian life, he assumed those experiences would translate easily into healthcare employment. Instead, he discovered that additional education was required to convert battlefield training into licensed clinical practice. Nursing became the bridge that allowed him to continue the work he felt most drawn to.

Returning to school after military service required a different kind of adjustment. Jason found that the academic structure of civilian education felt unfamiliar at first, particularly after years in operational environments where training was highly applied rather than lecture-focused. Yet the clinical portions of nursing school felt natural, reinforcing skills he had already practiced in high-intensity settings. Instructors often noted his calm demeanor during simulation exercises, especially scenarios involving rapid patient deterioration or trauma response. What had once been survival-driven field care now evolved into structured clinical practice supported by interdisciplinary hospital teams. Nursing expanded his role from emergency stabilization to ongoing patient management, communication with families, and coordination across multiple departments—responsibilities that required both technical skill and interpersonal communication.

By **06:15**, Jason was already driving toward the hospital, the early morning sky still dim as traffic gradually increased. His current role in the emergency department aligned closely with his previous experience, yet the environment differed in important ways. Hospital emergency care involved longer patient interactions, detailed documentation, and collaboration with a broader network of specialists than he had experienced in the field. Early in his transition, adjusting to these processes required patience, but he came to appreciate how coordinated systems improved continuity of care. Emergency departments demanded the same rapid prioritization he had learned in the military, but they also emphasized long-term recovery planning once immediate threats were stabilized. The combination of urgency and continuity gave the role a sense of completeness he had not expected.

Morning shift turnover at **06:58** brought the typical emergency department briefing: patient volumes trending upward overnight, several trauma cases expected from regional transport routes, and a staffing update outlining which clinicians were assigned to triage, fast-track, and high-acuity zones. Jason reviewed his assignment and began preparing supplies at his station, a habit developed during military service where readiness often determined response speed. Within the first hour, the department received a motor vehicle accident patient requiring immediate assessment and stabilization. Working alongside physicians, respiratory therapists, and fellow nurses, Jason assisted with rapid interventions while maintaining steady communication across the team. The pace felt familiar, yet the collaborative structure of the hospital setting added layers of coordination that made outcomes more predictable than the chaotic environments he had once known.

Late in the afternoon, the department quieted briefly between surges, giving Jason time to assist a newly hired nurse who was still adjusting to emergency department workflow. Mentorship had become one of the unexpected rewards of his transition into nursing. He understood how intimidating the first months in emergency care could feel and made a point of sharing practical strategies that helped maintain focus during high-pressure situations. Many former service members entering healthcare found similar fulfillment in teaching, recognizing that experience gained under difficult conditions could guide others entering the profession. The ability to pass forward lessons learned created a sense of continuity between past service and present career.

By **19:22**, after completing final documentation and shift handoff, Jason stepped outside into the evening air, the familiar post-shift fatigue settling in as the adrenaline of the day gradually faded. Driving home, he thought briefly about the uncertainty he once felt during his transition out of the military, unsure how his previous experience would translate into civilian work. Nursing had provided the pathway that allowed him to continue serving in a different form—protecting health rather than responding to conflict, yet still operating in environments where preparedness and teamwork mattered every day. As the city lights passed outside the windshield, he reflected on how the journey from medic to Registered Nurse had not erased his previous identity; it had expanded it. The mission had changed, but the purpose remained remarkably similar.

Journey 6 — The Burnout-to-Alignment Return

At **06:02**, the sunlight filtering through the apartment blinds arrived a few minutes before the alarm, and Rachel Nguyen, RN, BSN, stretched slowly before reaching for her phone. Unlike earlier in her career, mornings no longer began with a sense of dread. There had been a period—nearly two years—when she considered leaving nursing entirely, convinced that the exhaustion she felt meant the profession itself was the problem. Long shifts on a chronically understaffed unit had gradually eroded her enthusiasm, and the constant pressure to pick up extra hours made it difficult to recover between workdays. Friends outside healthcare often assumed burnout meant she needed a completely new career, yet what she eventually discovered was something different: sometimes the issue is not the profession, but the environment within it. Nursing had not changed; the conditions surrounding her role had.

Rachel's first years after graduation were spent on a fast-paced medical-surgical unit where the learning curve was steep and the patient volume consistently high. Initially, the challenge energized her, and she appreciated how quickly she developed clinical confidence. Over time, however, persistent staffing shortages and unpredictable scheduling created a cycle of fatigue that left little space for recovery. She began questioning whether she could realistically sustain the workload long term, especially as personal priorities outside work became more important. After speaking with mentors and former classmates working in other specialties, she realized she had been treating her current unit as the only version of nursing available. The profession, she learned, offered far more variety than she had initially explored.

By **06:40**, coffee finished brewing while Rachel reviewed the day's schedule—an outpatient procedural center shift that began at **08:00**, providing a routine far more predictable than her earlier inpatient roles. Transitioning to the outpatient environment had required cross-training and several weeks of onboarding, but the change reshaped her relationship with the profession. Procedures moved quickly, patient interactions were focused yet meaningful, and evening hours were typically free from last-minute admissions or emergency surges. The pace remained busy, but the structure allowed her to maintain a consistent routine that supported both professional performance and personal well-being. Nursing had not become easier; it had simply become better aligned with how she functioned best.

During the morning intake process, Rachel greeted patients arriving for scheduled procedures, reviewing histories, confirming medications, and preparing them for the clinical team. Many patients arrived nervous, unsure what to expect, and she found that calm explanations often made the greatest difference in their experience. Communication had always been one of her strengths, yet in previous high-volume inpatient roles she rarely had time to use it fully. The outpatient setting allowed those interpersonal skills to become a central part of her daily work rather than a rushed afterthought. Alignment, she realized, was not about finding a job without stress; it was about finding a role where her strengths were used consistently instead of occasionally. That difference alone restored a sense of professional satisfaction she thought she had lost.

By **14:10**, the procedural schedule moved steadily, patients rotating through preparation, procedure, and recovery areas in a coordinated rhythm. Rachel collaborated with physicians, anesthesia teams, and fellow nurses to ensure transitions remained smooth, stepping in wherever patient needs required additional support. The environment demanded efficiency, yet it also provided closure—patients typically left the same day, allowing nurses to see the complete arc of care rather than handing off cases mid-process. That sense of completion created a different kind of professional reward, one she had not anticipated earlier in her career. It reminded her that fulfillment in nursing often depends as much on setting selection as on the profession itself.

At **17:18**, after final documentation and shift wrap-up, Rachel stepped outside into the early evening light, noticing how different the end of the day felt compared with the exhaustion she once carried home from inpatient shifts. The work remained meaningful, but it no longer consumed every ounce of emotional and physical energy. Driving home, she reflected on how close she had come to leaving nursing entirely, not because she lacked ability or dedication, but because she had not yet discovered the specialty that fit her best. The experience changed how she now advises newer nurses: before deciding that nursing is not for you, consider whether the environment simply is not the right match. As she parked outside her apartment and gathered her bag, the realization felt simple but important—sometimes the path forward is not leaving the profession, but finding the place within it where you can finally stay.

Chapter 56

A Final Word on Momentum

Careers in nursing rarely unfold in perfectly predictable lines. Some years accelerate learning, others test endurance, and many quietly build the confidence that only experience can create. What matters most is not choosing a flawless starting point, but continuing to move forward with curiosity, adaptability, and a willingness to grow as the profession evolves. Each shift, each patient interaction, and each new responsibility gradually shapes clinical judgment in ways no classroom alone can provide. Stay engaged, stay reflective, and allow your career to develop one meaningful step at a time — momentum, not perfection, is what ultimately builds a lasting nursing career.

Chapter 57
Glossary

Glossary

Throughout this book, you encountered selected terms marked within the text to help familiarize you with the language commonly used across nursing practice, education, and healthcare environments. While no glossary can fully capture the complete vocabulary used in modern healthcare, the following reference section provides a working foundation of essential terminology that Registered Nurses encounter regularly in clinical communication, documentation, interdisciplinary collaboration, and patient education. Understanding these terms strengthens clinical clarity, reduces communication errors, and supports faster adaptation to real-world care settings where time-sensitive decisions rely on precise language.

Many of the words included here will appear repeatedly across specialties—whether in emergency care, surgical services, pediatrics, outpatient settings, or long-term care—while others may become more relevant as you move into specific practice areas or pursue advanced certifications. Healthcare language evolves alongside clinical innovation, but core terminology remains remarkably consistent across settings, making early familiarity an important professional advantage. Rather than attempting to memorize every term immediately, use this glossary as a return reference during training, clinical rotations, or early career transitions when unfamiliar terminology arises.

Over time, the vocabulary of nursing becomes second nature, allowing clinicians to focus less on translation and more on critical thinking, patient advocacy, and care coordination. Language fluency in healthcare is not about sounding technical; it is about ensuring that every member of the care team shares the same understanding at the exact moment clarity matters most.

Chapter 58

The 100 Words Every Registered Nurse Should Begin Learning

Healthcare speaks its own language. Walk into any hospital, clinic, or procedural center and you will quickly hear conversations filled with abbreviations, shorthand terminology, medication names, and clinical phrases that sound almost like a different dialect. For new nurses—and especially for students or readers still exploring the profession—this language can initially feel overwhelming, even intimidating. Yet learning the vocabulary of nursing is not about memorizing complex words for the sake of sounding clinical; it is about developing the communication fluency that allows care teams to move quickly, safely, and clearly in environments where time and precision matter. Shared terminology reduces confusion, strengthens teamwork, and ensures that important information travels accurately between clinicians, departments, and shifts.

The goal of this section is not to turn you into an expert overnight, but to introduce foundational terms you will encounter repeatedly across nursing education, clinical rotations, and early professional practice. Many of these words will appear in conversations between nurses, physicians, respiratory therapists, pharmacists, and other members of the care team, while others are commonly used in charting, patient education, or daily workflow communication. Becoming familiar with these terms early helps reduce the cognitive load that new clinicians often experience when trying to process unfamiliar language while simultaneously learning clinical skills. Vocabulary confidence creates mental space for critical thinking, and critical thinking is the foundation of safe patient care.

You will notice that some terms are highly technical, while others are deceptively simple phrases that carry very specific meanings within healthcare settings. Learning both types matters. Understanding terminology related to medications, diagnostics, patient status, and clinical procedures allows you to follow discussions more easily, ask clearer questions, and participate more confidently in patient-care coordination. Over time, this language becomes second nature, but early exposure significantly shortens the learning curve. Think of this glossary not as a test to study for, but as a toolkit you will return to repeatedly as your understanding grows.

As you move through the list, focus less on memorizing everything at once and more on recognizing patterns. Many medical terms share common prefixes, suffixes, and root meanings that make unfamiliar words easier to interpret once the building blocks are understood. The more you see and hear these terms in real contexts—during coursework, simulations, or clinical experiences—the more naturally they will become part of your professional vocabulary. Healthcare communication is fast-paced, but it is also structured, and learning its structure allows you to participate more effectively from the very beginning of your journey.

The following pages introduce **100 essential terms every Registered Nurse should begin learning**, serving as a practical language foundation that supports everything from classroom learning to bedside care.

1. Acute

A condition that begins suddenly and is often severe but typically short in duration.

2. Admission

The formal process of a patient being accepted into a hospital or healthcare facility for treatment.

3. Adverse Reaction

An unintended and harmful response to a medication or treatment.

4. Ambulate

To walk or assist a patient in walking for mobility and recovery purposes.

5. Analgesic

A medication used to relieve pain.

6. Assessment

The systematic evaluation of a patient's physical, emotional, and clinical condition.

7. Auscultation

Listening to internal body sounds, typically using a stethoscope, such as heart or lung sounds.

8. Baseline

The initial set of clinical measurements used as a reference point for future comparisons.

9. Bradycardia

A slower-than-normal heart rate, typically defined as fewer than 60 beats per minute in adults.

10. Catheter

A flexible tube inserted into the body to drain fluids or deliver medications.

11. Chronic

A condition that persists for a long time, often months or years.

12. Code Blue

An emergency alert indicating a patient requiring immediate resuscitation, often due to cardiac or respiratory arrest.

13. Contraindication

A factor or condition that makes a particular treatment or medication inappropriate or potentially harmful.

14. Culture (Lab Test)

A laboratory test used to identify microorganisms such as bacteria or fungi from a sample.

15. Dehydration

A condition in which the body loses more fluids than it takes in, leading to fluid imbalance.

16. Diagnosis

The identification of a disease or medical condition based on evaluation and testing.

17. Discharge

The formal release of a patient from a healthcare facility after treatment is completed.

18. Dyspnea

Difficulty or discomfort in breathing; shortness of breath.

19. Edema

Swelling caused by excess fluid trapped in body tissues.

20. Electrolytes

Minerals in the body fluids, such as sodium and potassium, that are essential for nerve and muscle function.

21. Fever

An elevated body temperature, often indicating infection or illness.

22. Hemorrhage

Excessive or uncontrolled bleeding.

23. Hypertension

Abnormally high blood pressure.

24. Hypoglycemia

Abnormally low blood sugar levels.

25. Infection

The invasion and multiplication of microorganisms in the body causing illness.

26. Infusion

The administration of fluids or medications directly into the bloodstream, typically through an intravenous (IV) line.

27. Intake

The total amount of fluids taken into the body, usually recorded as part of patient monitoring.

28. Isolation

Protective measures used to prevent the spread of infectious diseases within healthcare settings.

29. IV (Intravenous)

A method of delivering fluids or medications directly into a vein.

30. Lesion

An abnormal area of tissue that may result from injury, infection, or disease.

31. Medication Reconciliation

The process of reviewing and verifying a patient's medication list to ensure accuracy and safety.

32. Monitor

Equipment used to continuously observe a patient's vital signs or physiological activity.

33. NPO (Nothing by Mouth)

A medical instruction indicating that a patient should not eat or drink.

34. Oxygen Saturation

The percentage of oxygen carried by hemoglobin in the blood.

35. Pain Scale

A standardized tool used to measure the intensity of a patient's pain.

36. Palpation

The examination of the body by touch to assess structures or detect abnormalities.

37. Pathology

The study of diseases and the laboratory examination of tissues or bodily fluids.

38. Postoperative

The period following a surgical procedure.

39. Preoperative

The period before a surgical procedure.

40. Prognosis

The expected course or outcome of a disease or condition.

41. Pulse

The rhythmic expansion of arteries caused by heartbeats, measured to assess heart rate.

42. Recovery

The phase in which a patient regains strength or health after illness or surgery.

43. Respiratory Rate

The number of breaths taken per minute.

44. Sedation

The use of medication to calm a patient or induce sleep.

45. Specimen

A sample of tissue, blood, or other bodily material collected for laboratory analysis.

46. Sterile

Free from microorganisms, especially during medical procedures to prevent infection.

47. Sutures

Medical stitches used to close wounds or surgical incisions.

48. Tachycardia

An abnormally fast heart rate, typically over 100 beats per minute in adults.

49. Triage

The process of prioritizing patients based on the severity of their condition.

50. Vital Signs

Key clinical measurements—temperature, pulse, respiratory rate, blood pressure, and sometimes oxygen saturation—used to assess patient status.

51. Wound Care

The treatment and management of injuries to promote healing and prevent infection.

52. Allergic Reaction

An immune-system response to a substance that the body identifies as harmful.

53. Anticoagulant

A medication that helps prevent blood clot formation.

54. Antibiotic

A medication used to treat bacterial infections.

55. Arrhythmia

An abnormal heart rhythm that may be too fast, too slow, or irregular.

56. Aspiration

The inhalation of food, liquid, or other material into the lungs.

57. Biopsy

The removal of a small tissue sample for laboratory examination.

58. Blood Glucose

The level of sugar present in the bloodstream.

59. Cardiac Output

The amount of blood the heart pumps each minute.

60. Compression

The application of pressure to control bleeding or reduce swelling.

61. Contusion

A bruise caused by injury to blood vessels under the skin.

62. Defibrillator

A device used to deliver an electric shock to restore a normal heart rhythm.

63. Dehiscence

The reopening of a surgical incision or wound.

64. Drainage

Fluid that flows from a wound, incision, or body cavity.

65. Dressing

Protective material placed over a wound to promote healing.

66. Dysphagia

Difficulty swallowing.

67. Endoscopy

A procedure using a flexible instrument to view the inside of the body.

68. Fatigue

A state of extreme tiredness or exhaustion.

69. Fracture

A break in a bone.

70. Gait

A person's manner of walking.

71. Hemoglobin

The protein in red blood cells responsible for carrying oxygen.

72. Immunization

The process of becoming protected against disease through vaccination.

73. Incision

A surgical cut made in the body.

74. Inflammation

The body's response to injury or infection, often causing redness, swelling, and pain.

75. Intramuscular (IM)

A method of injecting medication directly into a muscle.

76. Intradermal (ID)

A method of injecting medication just beneath the surface of the skin.

77. Intrathecal

Medication administered into the spinal canal.

78. Laceration

A deep cut or tear in the skin or tissue.

79. Leukocytes

White blood cells that help fight infection.

80. Malignant

A term used to describe cancerous cells that can spread to other parts of the body.

81. Metastasis

The spread of cancer cells from one part of the body to another.

82. Necrosis

The death of body tissue caused by lack of blood supply, infection, or injury.

83. Neurological Assessment

Evaluation of the nervous system, including consciousness, movement, and reflexes.

84. Nutrition Support

Medical methods used to provide nutrients when a patient cannot eat normally.

85. Orthostatic Hypotension

A drop in blood pressure that occurs when standing up from sitting or lying down.

86. Palliative Care

Medical care focused on relieving symptoms and improving quality of life for patients with serious illness.

87. Percutaneous

A procedure performed through the skin.

88. Perfusion

The flow of blood through body tissues and organs.

89. Platelets

Blood components that help with clotting.

90. Polyuria

Excessive urination.

91. Pressure Ulcer

An injury to skin and underlying tissue caused by prolonged pressure.

92. Rehabilitation

Therapy designed to restore strength, mobility, or function after illness or injury.

93. Remission

A period during which symptoms of a disease decrease or disappear.

94. Sepsis

A life-threatening condition caused by the body's response to infection.

95. Shock

A critical condition where the body is not receiving adequate blood flow.

96. Thrombosis

The formation of a blood clot inside a blood vessel.

97. Transfusion

The transfer of blood or blood products into the bloodstream.

98. Ulcer

An open sore on the skin or internal lining of the body.

99. Ventilation

The movement of air into and out of the lungs, sometimes assisted by mechanical devices.

100. Withdrawal

The process of gradually reducing or stopping medications or substances to prevent adverse effects.

Chapter 59

The Never End

Every career journey has moments that feel like endings — graduation days, first jobs, specialty transitions, or the closing of one chapter before another begins. Yet in healthcare, very few moments are true endings. Each experience becomes preparation for the next responsibility, the next skill, the next opportunity to serve patients and communities in new ways. Nursing, perhaps more than most professions, evolves alongside the person practicing it. Roles change, specialties shift, priorities grow, and new pathways appear that were not visible at the beginning. What may feel like the end of one stage is usually the beginning of another, often one that brings greater clarity, confidence, and purpose.

This is the idea behind *The Never End*: your career does not move in a straight line toward a single destination. Instead, it unfolds as a series of evolving chapters, each building upon the last. The experiences you gain in one unit, one specialty, or one season of life often become the skills that open doors later — into leadership, education, advanced practice, community care, or entirely new clinical environments. Even the challenges that feel most difficult in the moment frequently become the lessons that strengthen long-term professional resilience. Growth in healthcare is rarely instant, but it is remarkably continuous for those who remain open to learning and adapting.

If this book has helped you better understand what Registered Nurse practice truly involves — the responsibilities, the realities, the opportunities, and the decisions ahead — then it has served its purpose. Whether you are preparing to enter nursing, exploring specialty directions, or evaluating the next step in your professional path, the most important decision you can make is choosing a role that aligns with how you work best and where you can sustain your energy over time. Alignment does not eliminate hard days, but it ensures that the work remains meaningful enough to continue.

Healthcare needs skilled professionals, but it also needs professionals who remain engaged long enough to grow into the leaders, mentors, and innovators the system depends upon. Your journey through nursing, wherever it leads, contributes to that larger story. And no matter which direction your path takes next, remember that the profession offers more routes forward than most people realize. What feels like a final step today may simply be the opening of another door tomorrow.

Goodbye for now,

Mason Preddy

Mason Preddy

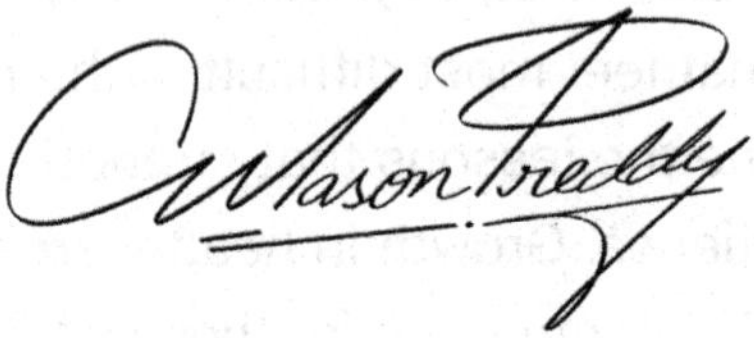

Chapter 60

About the Author

Mason Preddy is a healthcare workforce strategist, publisher, and career-alignment advocate with more than 2.5 decades of experience in healthcare recruitment, retention strategy, and workforce consulting across hospitals, academic medical centers, specialty practices, and national healthcare organizations. Over the course of his career, he has worked closely with clinical leaders, executives, educators, and frontline professionals to better understand the forces shaping healthcare career satisfaction, burnout trends, and long-term workforce sustainability. His work focuses on helping healthcare professionals choose roles that align with their strengths, career goals, and life priorities—an approach designed to improve both retention and long-term professional fulfillment.

As the founder of **Mason Maison™ Publishing**, Preddy leads the development of career-navigation resources that translate real-world workforce insights into accessible guidance for students, early-career clinicians, and experienced professionals exploring new directions. His flagship career-alignment framework integrates workforce data, behavioral career insights, and lived-experience narratives to help readers make informed decisions before committing to demanding professional pathways. Through the *ScrubTales™* series and related career-assessment tools, his work emphasizes a central principle: healthcare careers are most sustainable when professional roles match how individuals are naturally wired to work, communicate, and manage responsibility.

Preddy continues to collaborate with healthcare leaders, educators, and workforce organizations to expand access to alignment-focused career planning tools for the next generation of healthcare professionals. His publishing initiatives support students, clinicians, and institutions seeking practical guidance on career fit, specialty selection, long-term growth pathways, and the evolving realities of modern healthcare practice.

Chapter 61

Also by Mason Maison™ Publishing

What Color Are Your Scrubs?™ — The Complete Healthcare Career Guide

A comprehensive career-navigation resource introducing more than 340 healthcare professions across clinical, technical, leadership, and support roles. Designed to help students, career changers, and healthcare professionals explore pathways before committing to education or specialty training, the guide integrates real-world workforce insights, alignment-based decision frameworks, and practical planning strategies to support long-term career sustainability.

SCRUB*fit*™ Healthcare Career Assessment

A structured career-alignment assessment tool designed to help individuals evaluate personality fit, work-style preferences, environmental needs, and long-term career sustainability within healthcare professions. The assessment complements the career-navigation framework introduced in

What Color Are Your Scrubs?™ and supports more targeted exploration of specialty pathways and training decisions.

ScrubTales™ Career Series

A growing series of specialty-specific healthcare career guides providing in-depth, real-world insights into individual professions across the healthcare landscape. Each volume explores daily practice realities, hiring systems, compensation structures, specialty pathways, and long-term career mobility while incorporating cinematic day-in-the-life narratives that illustrate how each role functions in real clinical environments.

Made in the USA
Monee, IL
05 November 2026

67911935R00167